QUESTIONS AND ANSWERS
ON FAMILY HEALTH

Questions and Answers on Family Health

The Alternative Approach

Foreword by
Dr Alfred Vogel

Jan de Vries

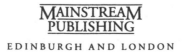

MAINSTREAM
PUBLISHING

EDINBURGH AND LONDON

First published in Great Britain in 1994 by
MAINSTREAM PUBLISHING COMPANY (EDINBURGH) LTD
7 Albany Street
Edinburgh EH1 3UG

Reprinted 1997, 1999

ISBN 1 85158 586 9 (cloth)
ISBN 1 85158 587 7 (paper)

A catalogue record for this book is available from the British Library

Typeset in Perpetua by Litholink Ltd, Welshpool
Printed and bound by WSOY, Finland

Contents

Foreword

It was a fortunate occasion when I met Jan de Vries in January 1959 in the Netherlands. I spoke to him with pleasure and conviction about my 40 years' experience in the field of herbal medicine and my views on diet and nourishment. I soon realised that I had an extremely interested listener who fully appreciated my knowledge of the whole sphere of medical science.

Jan de Vries was not only interested to learn everything about my experiences of when, where and how to collect herbs, he also insisted on taking part in the actual process of extracting their beneficial ingredients. As he was a trained and qualified pharmacist, he was already familiar with the world of plants and herbs and had considerable knowledge in this field. He accepted an invitation to join our firm, which gave us the chance to establish a working relationship which has lasted for many years. He was one of my best pupils, if not the very best, and he grasped the opportunity to further develop his talents in the field of natural medicine.

I was very happy to share with him my enthusiasm for Nature and the world of plants. He was also prepared to accept my principle that herbal medicine should always have priority in the treatment of illness.

As a result of our experiences we both agreed that, when properly used, natural methods and herbal remedies could improve one's health and keep illnesses at bay. Nature itself is capable of healing. Jan de Vries shared my conviction that herbal medicine in combination with a natural diet could create positive responses in the body in order to ward off ailments. By creating the right conditions for the body and supplying it with the correct nourishment, we are able to activate the body's own regeneration system. In this way it is possible to overcome, as well as cure, ailments. Natural practitioners are becoming increasingly aware that we don't just have an important role to play in the curing of illnesses, but also in the prevention of medical disturbances. This requires us to put greater emphasis on preventive medicine. Prevention is always better than cure.

This principle plays a major role in my own approach. In an effort to clarify this to patients and the public at large, I have written several books, such as *The Nature Doctor*, *The Liver as the Regulator of our Health*, and *Nature, Your Guide to Healthier Living*.

Jan de Vries was immediately prepared to share my experiences with his friends and later with his patients and he recommended these books for their information. He is, I am pleased to repeat, my most successful 'pupil'. His success, from which many patients have benefited is not, however, attributable solely to his talents; it is also thanks to the Creator who has supplied so many plants with healing powers.

I am very pleased that Jan de Vries is able to share his knowledge and experiences with us on paper. His books are written in simple language that can be readily understood by both patients and laymen alike. In these books he deals with natural methods using herbal remedies to overcome ailments and illnesses.

It is important to look beyond merely curing the obvious symptoms, as conventional medicine might teach us. We must look for the cause of the illness in order to continue the treatment and find a cure for the source. Very little benefit is obtained by clearing up an ache or easing a sensitivity if we are not able to eliminate the cause. In order to do this we should study the whole person and attempt to recognise which factors have contributed to the condition. There could be many reasons, for example, a breathing difficulty, a movement disorder, or a shortage of oxygen, rest or sleep. There can be many causes of a biological imbalance.

Jan de Vries has developed an extensive knowledge in this area. With perseverance he builds up an overall picture of total health, never failing to take into account the physical and mental condition of the patient.

I am convinced that in this book he will show many people the right way to recovery in plain and simple language. It is an excellent complement to my own books, as we have both sincerely attempted to serve our fellow men and share with them the knowledge we have acquired from our understanding and experience of the bounty of nature.

Dr Alfred Vogel

Introduction

Questions and Answers on Family Health is the handbook for every household and has been published in direct response to public demand. During the hundreds of lectures that I have given throughout the world over the years, at conferences and public meetings, I often asked for the questions to be written down so that I could answer them from the platform. I kept many of these questions with the intention at the back of my mind of possibly collating them at a later time into a compilation for the interested reader. The infinite variety of topics covered by these questions gives a fair impression of the public's interest in and approach towards Alternative Medicine. Some interesting questions from the many radio and television broadcasts I have participated in, especially the well-known Gloria Hunniford BBC Radio 2 series, have also been incorporated in this book.

It often seems that books on similar subjects contradict each other, and the questions from meetings and lectures are a good indicator of what the public wants to know and learn about. These questions may be so diverse as to cover varicose veins, the use of vitamin E, headaches, verrucas, ME, *Candida*, or cancer. The health problems and concerns experienced by people today are so numerous that it is impossible to assemble them all into one publication. However, this handbook presents a variety of easily used methods and I have tried to keep the contents as useful and varied as possible.

It is my sincere wish that this book will be of help to a great many people and that its readers will find the answers to some of their own questions in this book.

The reader should bear in mind that any advice, remedy or method mentioned in this book, is suggested as a guideline only. I would always recommend that people consult a qualified practitioner for specific advice.

A

ABSCESSES

How can I avoid an abscess recurring?

An abscess can be an extremely uncomfortable and often painful affliction. It is generally regarded as an accumulation of internal and external toxic material and indicates a high level of toxicity in the body. Although the lymphatic system collects and disposes of most of the body's waste material, sometimes it may not be able to cope with excessive demands. Excessive toxicity in the body is often the result of an unbalanced or unsuitable diet, exacerbated by alcohol and/or nicotine.

I would recommend Echinaforce (15 drops in some water before meals, taken twice daily), Petaforce (ten drops in a little water before meals, taken twice daily) and two tablets of *Hepar sulph. 4x* before going to bed.

I suffer from recurring abscesses for which my doctor prescribes antibiotics. I would like to know if there is a homoeopathic alternative?

In the case of recurring abscesses one should first of all look at the diet. Do not eat fatty foods and ban all pork and pork derivatives e.g. pork chops, bacon, ham, etc. Avoid spices, alcohol and nicotine. Eat plenty of fruit and vegetables. Take ten drops of Petaforce in half a cup of water twice a day. You would also be well advised to use garlic or a garlic-based product. For centuries garlic has been used as a dietary constituent and it is a common ingredient of Mediterranean dishes. In Britain alone, in excess of one hundred million garlic capsules are purchased every year. Researchers are now beginning to accept that it possesses remarkable effective powers: apart from its benefits to the digestive system, natural garlic may help to maintain normal cholesterol levels in the blood, when used as part of a healthy low-fat diet.

ACNE

What is the cause of acne?
There are two common kinds of acne: acne vulgaris and acne rosacea. As
the name indicates, the first is more common, and it is also easier to treat.
Acne vulgaris is an inflammatory condition of the sebaceous glands in the
skin, mostly affecting the face, neck, chest and back. The exact cause of
acne cannot be determined, but it is often thought to result from a
hormonal imbalance, which is why teenagers in particular tend to
experience this problem. Hereditary influences can also play a role and
certain foods have been known to aggravate the condition. Therefore the
first rule in treating acne vulgaris is to adopt a healthy diet.

Acne rosacea, however, presents a much bigger problem as it is
generally more difficult to control. This is a chronic skin condition
affecting the fleshy areas of the face, the nose, cheeks, chin and forehead,
which affects both sexes, usually in middle age. This condition is thought
to be caused by neurovascular instability, endocrine disorders, allergies and
various other factors. The first requirement, once again, is a healthy diet.

The following remedies are recommended for both types of acne:
Echinaforce, *Viola tricolor*, Petaforce, vitamin E and Oil of Evening
Primrose.

**What diet, juices and herbs do you recommend for persistent
acne? I have tried almost everything.**
Drink plenty of beetroot and carrot juice and take Dr Vogel's
Violaforce. Also follow this general diet:

Diet for acne sufferers
Breakfast
Vogel's Breakfast Muesli mixed with the juice of a grated apple or half a
banana or other fruit (no citrus fruits).
One or two pieces of Ryvita or wholemeal bread spread with natural
vegetable magarine (sunflower or corn-oil margarine).
One cup of tea after the meal, preferably peppermint, rosehip or
camomile tea. Bambu coffee may be used as an alternative.

Lunch
One plate of fresh vegetables, especially carrots and beetroot. Some other

raw or cooked vegetables. Dress the fresh vegetables with olive or sunflower oil mixed with a little lemon juice or celery juice.

Baked or steamed potatoes in their jackets may be taken with the vegetables.

For dessert, take natural unflavoured yogurt, sweetened with honey if desired.

Dinner

Vegetable soup made with fresh, organically grown vegetables. The water used to prepare the soup can be enriched with a little Plantaforce; this is a delicious vegetable concentrate from the Vogel range and is very easily digested. Use salt sparingly in this soup – a little Herbamare is more beneficial.

Fresh fruit salad may be taken for dessert, although if you are prone to indigestion, do not combine these two.

General advice

Animal fat is prohibited. Use eggs sparingly. No white flour or white sugar (or products made with them). No pork, sausages, bacon or ham. Cut down as much as possible on coffee, nicotine and sweets. Take plenty of exercise in the fresh air.

Please advise on treatment for acne in a teenage boy.

Give the boy one capsule of AkneZyme twice daily.

My daughter has acne. She took antibiotics for six months and it went away. She stopped taking the antibiotics and it came back. The doctor recently again prescribed antibiotics: Minocrin MR, which was accompanied by a warning about possible side-effects. For the first few weeks my daughter was all right, but during the last two weeks she has had very severe (thumping) headaches and sometimes cannot bear to see bright lights. My daughter wants to go back to her GP, but I would like to ask you if you have a safe way of treating acne?

In short, my answer is *yes*! This problem can be approached from several different angles and therefore I would suggest that you and your daughter read my book *Skin Disorders*, which gives details on various treatment approaches.

Can homoeopathic medicine help acne sufferers?
It most certainly can. Please read my book *Skin Disorders* for advice on a wide variety of alternative treatment methods for acne, and also for other skin complaints.

I have suffered from acne since I was a teenager. I am now 37. I have tried nearly all the treatments available on NHS. Can you help?
Read up on the dietary advice you can find in this section. You may like to consider acupuncture treatment, which is often helpful.

ANAEMIA

How do I overcome anaemia?
Anaemia is a condition characterised by a reduced number of red blood corpuscles or of haemoglobin in the bloodstream, which in turn reduces the blood's effectiveness in transporting oxygen throughout the body. It identifies itself by the patient's lack of energy and general listlessness, and is caused by a lack of iron.

Pernicious anaemia is a specific form of anaemia and, fortunately, less common than the type described above. This condition is characterised by lesions of the spinal cord, weakness, diarrhoea, a sore tongue and numbness in the limbs. It is usually associated with an inadequate absorption of vitamin B^{12}. In addition to the recommended medication, diet is very important. Supplement a balanced diet three times a week with a dessert of four dried pears (sulphur-free) soaked in red grape juice or port wine. Eat plenty of fresh green vegetables and a raw egg, beaten with red grape juice about three times a week. Use Alfavena tablets, *Ferrum phos. 6x* and *Kalium phos. 6x.*

ADDICTIONS
Alcohol
In our society it is considered socially acceptable to 'have a drink'. I can put it more strongly, the person who does not take a drink is, often derogatively, labelled a 'teetotaller'. Yet, what is mostly seen as a pleasant social custom too often gets out of hand and ends in abuse. Acupuncture

can help to overcome alcohol dependence, in combination with the following remedies: brewers' yeast (4-6 tablets per day) and vitamin C (up to 2 g daily).

Nicotine

Not so long ago it was considered socially acceptable to smoke wherever one liked. Fortunately, this attitude has now reversed and not before time. Today, smokers complain that they are treated as outcasts, but they should remember that indulgence pollutes the surrounding atmosphere. Non-smokers are forced to breathe in stale air and therefore have to partake in a habit which is far from conducive to their health. As with alcohol addiction, this habit is equally difficult to break, but again acupuncture treatment can be helpful together with a homoeopathic nicotine substitute, *Tabacum 4x*. Five drops should be taken twice daily in a little water.

Sugar

This addiction not only causes the obvious weight problems, but it also affects the condition of the skin. Gradually reducing the sugar intake is the best approach, in order to avoid a shock to the system and this can be helped with Oil of Evening Primrose (three capsules taken last thing at night) and ginseng.

ALLERGIES

Why are there so many allergies?
An allergy is an abnormal sensitivity to a specific substance. Not only is it possible to become allergic to certain foods, but also to atmospheric influences, pollutants or pollen for example. If our reserves were strong enough and if we paid more attention to leading a life according to the laws of Nature and investing sensibly in our health, there would be fewer allergies. An allergy only becomes obvious when a person's immune system allows it to do so. A developing allergic trend is, in effect, no more than an alarm bell, an early warning that the immune system is struggling to protect the body against outside influences and is becoming less effective. Pay attention to these alarm signals and remember that the root cause should be treated, rather than the symptom. Concentrate on

revitalising the immune system and often the allergy will disappear of its own accord.

What causes allergies? Too often the recommended treatment seems to be aimed at relieving the symptoms and I wonder if they can be overcome by restoring positive and negative harmony?
This can only be achieved by boosting and re-building the immune system.

My sister was stung by a wasp last Thursday. She fainted and woke up in hospital, where she was kept under observation for two days. Is there anything you can suggest so that this does not happen again?
Your sister should use *Harpagophytum* and also follow a good blood-cleansing programme. Read my book *Viruses, Allergies and the Immune System* for further advice.

I would like to find out what foods I am allergic to, but this seems to be an insurmountable problem if the allergies are likely to vary, even within short periods of time.
We must remember that if our diet is balanced and healthy, our immune system will be stronger. If our diet is inadequate, we must take dietary supplements such as vitamins, minerals and trace elements to reduce the chance of allergic reactions.

Can an allergy to dairy products induce hyperactivity in a three-year-old who was allergic to dairy produce as a baby?
This is most unusual, as at that age it is more likely that hyperactivity is caused by excessive sugar intake.

Can one become allergic to *Echinacea* or Echinaforce?
In my experience this is most unlikely as *Echinacea* and Echinaforce are remedies that help to restore the immune system.

My friend was prescribed two homoeopathic remedies – *Harpagophytum* and Echinaforce (she is an artist and has a paint allergy which causes her to cough a lot). For how long should she take these remedies and when can she expect to notice an improvement?

Your friend would be well advised to continue with these remedies for a period of at least three months. The improvement in her condition will be gradual, as these remedies are designed to strengthen the immune system.

My wife has many environmental sensitivities and is now trying to detoxify her system. Does this carry any risk?
No, this is a very sensible approach. A very good detoxification programme is Dr Vogel's Detox Box Programme.

My son is allergic to fish and therefore eats a lot of meat. Is his diet incomplete?
I must point out that soya is also a good substitute for meat. Also ensure that his diet contains plenty of vegetables, fruit and nuts.

I suffer from a total allergy to all antibiotics and painkillers. What do you recommend I do for self-help?
There are alternative remedies that you can use and I would suggest that you seek the help of a qualified naturopath or homoeopath for the correct remedies for specific purposes.

What can be done for a child who is affected by 'E' colouring/additives in food?
No other measures are necessary than to avoid any products which contain 'E' colouring additives. Read the labels when shopping.

I am 62 years old and weigh approximately 10 stones. I drink raw garlic and fresh raspberry tea with a little Epsom salts. I also take garlic pills and cayenne pepper. I eat as many vegetables and fruit as possible, whole grains, etc. I am bothered with allergies in summer. What would you advise?
Although the remedies you take are good, they are not actually effective as an anti-allergy measure. Try 15 drops of *Harpagophytum* in a little water and two tablets of Imuno-Strength, both twice daily.

Could you comment on the relationship between inflammatory pain and wheat? The Homoeopathic Hospital believes that a wheat-free diet helps, but I am unconvinced.

In cases of a genuine wheat allergy, this substance can certainly cause inflammatory pains. You should try a wheat-free diet to see if the pains subside, but you must persevere for at least three months before you decide whether it is worthwhile.

I have chronic catarrh and I think it is because of an allergy. Can you suggest how I can remedy this?
Only too often I have seen this symptom caused by a dairy food allergy. This usually results in bad congestion. Try eliminating dairy food from your diet.

If one is allergic to something, could it be something that one enjoys especially?
Unfortunately, this is very often the case.

Can you suggest a simple method of testing for allergies?
Probably muscle-testing, known as Kinesiology.

Our mouths are full of metal fillings. What can we do to replace them? What substance should be used to fill our dental cavities?
The best idea is to gradually have all amalgam fillings removed and replaced with composite fillings, but during this period you and your family should take 20 drops of Echinaforce in a little water twice a day.

Could you explain how to detect an allergy to a certain food?
Allergy testing can done at home and in many cases people have been successful by following a food-elimination programme.

My daughter is allergic to homoeopathic tablets because of the lactose in them. She also seems to be allergic to the tincture. Is there another form these remedies can be taken in?
Usually, a fresh plant extract is best. If allergic to alcohol, put the remedy in hot water so that the alcohol evaporates.

What is the best natural anti-allergy medicine?
For the majority of cases I would suggest taking twenty drops of *Harpagophytum* twice daily in half a cup of water.

What would you recommend for a hay fever allergy?
This is an allergy to pollen. Dr Vogel's Pollinosan is generally beneficial. As far as diet is concerned, try to cut out all dairy foods and salt. Eat plenty of honey.

What does the body attempt to accomplish by sneezing?
Unusually frequent or excessive sneezing is the body's reaction to an allergic condition. Seek professional help.

How can I find out which food or drink triggers IBS (irritable bowel syndrome)?
In my experience the most common causes are coffee, stress or nerves, or a combination of these.

My son is extremely allergic to milk and eggs, which we discovered when he was weaned from the breast at the age of seven months. At 18 months old he was hospitalised for four days with asthma. He takes medication daily for asthma and allergies. Also, at the age of six he still has occasional incontinence. What can help him?
Most allergies do not occur until the baby is weaned and given cow's milk. The latter contains nine times more protein that mother's milk and the baby's digestive system cannot always cope. Infantile eczema and asthmatic attacks often occur then. For more detailed advice I suggest you read my book *Viruses, Allergies and the Immune System*.

I think I have allergies because my symptoms are congestion, a sore throat, ear infections, fatigue, body aches and ulcers. What can I do?
The best advice I could give you is to make an appointment with a homoeopath or naturopath. If preferred, follow a sensible detoxification programme such as The Detox Box Programme. Cleansing Course.

Is there something to be done for the dark rings under my eyes? I know that I have allergies.
You may have an allergy, but this is not necessarily the cause of your problem. It might also be a sign of kidney problems. Speak to your GP or see a naturopath.

What can someone do who is allergic to all medication?
Follow a desensitising programme.

Is it true that you can crave foods or other substances that you are allergic to?
Yes! Look at a migraine sufferer who is allergic to chocolate. He or she will always indulge when free of migraine.

Do mercury dental fillings cause disorders and, if so, can this be reversed?
Apart from gradually replacing these fillings, I would suggest that you follow a total detoxification programme.

How safe are mercury fillings?
It depends on the immune system. Preferably I would advise to have them replaced with composite fillings.

Can a severe allergy to peanut butter (such as my grandson has) be cured by your methods? The doctor has said that he could die within minutes of eating peanuts.
It all depends on what substance in peanut butter he is allergic to. First of all he needs a very thorough allergy test and based on the results of this a suitable treatment method can be selected.

ANOREXIA

Can you give some advice on how to overcome anorexia?
Twice a day take ten drops of *Centaurium umbellatum* in a little water before meals. Supplementary zinc and Nature's Best's Health Insurance Plus can be helpful too.

Can you give us any ideas on how we can help and support our daughter, who has anorexia?
Please read my book *Stress and Nervous Disorders*, where I have written about this illness in detail.

ANXIETY

Can you recommend a cure for anxiety?
Take, twice daily, ten drops of the Dr Vogel remedy Crataegus in a little water. Also take *Arsenicun album 4x* and *Strophanthus hispidus 4x*. For further help read my book *Stress and Nervous Disorders*.

Could you help a person who suffers from anxiety and nervous problems, e.g. fear of meeting people, and who also has difficulty in relaxing?
Take 15 drops of *Avena sativa* and two Jayvee tablets, both twice daily.

ARTHRITIS AND RHEUMATISM

Can you give an explanation of arthritis or rheumatism?
This cannot be done in a few lines and as these are such common disorders I will go into more detail. Swollen fingers, enlarged and twisted knuckles, swelling of the knees with fluid, a stiffened neck and spine – these conditions paint a terrible picture. Yet they are a familiar sight all around us. Severe and prolonged periods of pain make movement, sitting and sleeping difficult, and the only general relief is some pain-killing drug, which after a while has less and less effect. Cortisone is often prescribed, but does it produce a cure? No, because once such treatment commences, it is generally necessary 'for life'. Despite the large sums of money spent on research, there is still no cure available.

In the field of alternative medicine, however, more success is being achieved. The application of homoeopathic or herbal therapies is producing some remarkable results. These, along with the serious study of the relationship between diet and these illnesses, have shown that it is possible to bring considerable relief to those who suffer from these depressing symptoms. It is now generally accepted that although some people may inherit tendencies towards certain ailments, faulty diet greatly contributes towards producing illnesses like arthritis and rheumatism. In his book *The Nature Doctor* Dr Alfred Vogel says that 'The diet for arthritis and rheumatism should be absolutely natural. It should exclude acid-forming foods, in particular pork and processed meats.' He continues: 'It must be our faulty way of eating and living that accounts for the problems that we bring upon ourselves, because these diseases do not exist among the more primitive people.'

Additionally, acupuncture has proved valuable in stimulating the body functions, helping the body to remove the underlying causes of arthritis and rheumatism. It is therefore well worth everyone who suffers from these and related problems to seriously consider 'alternative' therapies.

We use the terms arthritis and rheumatism, but pain and limitation are what people actually experience. What are the events in our bodies that lead to such conditions developing? One factor that acts as a trigger is stress, that is anything and everything that threatens or damages us – fear, a heavy workload, the kind of food we eat. Although some stress is avoidable (for example we can stop smoking), we must all learn to cope with it in some form.

We can learn to live with stress. Physically, we must learn to replace the resources that we use. Our nutrition therefore has to be very good. There is a tiny gland at the base of the brain called the pituitary gland. At any sign of stress, this gland releases a hormone which sounds the alarm. The hormone travels in the blood until it reaches two small glands that sit on our kidneys in the middle of the back – the adrenals. When the adrenals pick up this hormone they too release different hormones. The better known of these is called cortisol (we know it as cortisone). Messages will have reached the adrenals from the nervous system too, and the hormone adrenalin is also released. The presence of these adrenal hormones in the blood tells the whole body that it is under threat.

The reaction is dramatic. Sugar reserves pour into the blood to provide immediate fuel. Proteins and fats are broken down to give more energy. Calcium is taken from our bones for use by the nerves and muscles. Pain, stiffness and inflammation seem to miraculously disappear. Blood pressure rises so that oxygen, sugar and calcium travel more quickly to the tissues.

The stress reaction is highly protective. Normally, the threat ends and the above reactions are gradually reversed. Proteins are rebuilt and the cells are repaired. Calcium is replaced in our bones. Blood pressure drops to its normal level and all our familiar aches and pains reappear. The body's reserves will have been used and even more will be needed for repair. More vitamins, minerals, protein, fats and carbohydrates will be needed than usual. When our nutrition is inadequate, or when the stress situation does not come to an end, our body will come under further threat. By robbing Peter to pay Paul, it will do the best it can for as long as it can. But sooner or later we will find we have no more reserves, we stop manufacturing adrenal hormones, and we have no further resistance. Disease is the result.

The removal of calcium from the bones when under stress is clearly one feature of the arthritic process. Normally, calcium moves continuously between blood and bone to maintain a balance. A hormone from the parathyroid gland in the neck triggers the removal of calcium from the bones when the blood level drops. Calcitonin, a hormone from the thyroid gland, encourages calcium back to the bone. Vitamins are needed for us to absorb calcium from our food and also to help the bone to mineralise. The balance of calcium is very delicate. If the blood levels drop, our muscles may go into spasms and convulsions. If our bones are continuously leached, they may bend or break. If the level of calcium in the blood stays high, as in a stressful condition, then calcium may be deposited in the arteries, tissues, muscles and joints. This depositing tendency appears to be an error resulting from prolonged stress without adequate nutrition, a parathyroid imbalance or vitamin deficiency.

The adrenals produce cortisol from the hormone deoxycortisol (known as DOC for short). This hormone has a remarkable action. It helps the body to fight infection and damage by setting up inflammation around bacteria or toxins and sealing them off, as in boils for example. Swelling, pain and fever may result but the body is being protected nonetheless. Normally, sufficient DOC will be converted to cortisol to remove the pain and swelling once the intruder has been dealt with.

When a diet does not supply the vitamins needed by the enzymes that make and maintain the balance of these hormones, the DOC may fail to be converted to cortisol and the areas of pain and swelling may become permanent and collect calcium. Cortisone treatment is not the easy solution because our own DOC production is inhibiting resistance. Our bones become further demineralised and other mineral reactions may cause water retention (moon face). Moreover, the constant robbing of proteins may eat away our stomach cells and cause ulcers.

The whole vitamin spectrum must be used when the nutrition pattern has broken down so severely. Other aspects of our diets must also be changed. When we eat sugar our blood sugar level rises rapidly and we feel full of energy, which is why we like it. Another gland, the pancreas, is alerted and insulin is released to absorb the sugar and store it. When we eat sugar frequently, our pancreas becomes trigger-happy and takes out too much at a time. We then develop low blood sugar, or hyperglycaemia.

The adrenals are alerted and we go into a stress reaction. Calcium is taken from our bones. So, when we eat sugar we can make holes in our bones, not just in our teeth.

Moreover, few of us realise we are addicted to salt. Salt is a stimulant: it hits the adrenals and once again we go into a stress reaction. Most of us eat ten times too much salt in a day because we like the 'high' it provides. The blood is naturally 80 per cent alkaline. The alkaline-forming foods are mainly fruit and vegetables, yogurt and seeds. If we eat an all-acid meal such as an egg on toast with coffee, the body's reserves of calcium and other minerals are drawn upon in order to restore the alkaline balance. As it is difficult to heal arthritis or rheumatism with an acid body, our food intake therefore should be 80 per cent alkaline and 20 per cent acid. Calcium must be added to the diet during the healing programme. The bones will only remineralise when there is sufficient in the diet.

Calcium enters into solution in an acid medium and is precipitated and deposited in an alkaline medium. This simple but profound statement provides the key to unlock the mystery of arthritis. To reverse this process – one of solubility – we must employ a secondary agent. This agent is potassium.

Rich sources of potassium are potatoes, molasses, bananas, cider vinegar, dates, apricots, figs and raisins. The enemies of potassium include alcohol, laxatives, coffee, sugar, salt and stress.

When treating every type of arthritis or rheumatism, the patient's diet has to be altered from a poor sub-nutritive diet to a rich energy-producing diet that is particularly rich in potassium. Potassium deficiency can produce rapid calcification of the arteries, teeth, muscles and joints. A diet low in potassium causes types of arthritis which are preceded by rheumatic disorders – aching muscles first and fixed joints afterwards. Finally, herbs are traditional cleansers and healers. As well as providing many vitamins and minerals themselves, the herbs used to treat these conditions work on all levels to help bring the body, mind and emotions back into healing alignment.

Can rheumatism and arthritis be successfully treated at home? The answer is *Yes* and a very good start may be achieved by keeping to the instructions outlined below. The treatment would be better still with the help and guidance of a qualified practitioner.

Programme for arthritis and rheumatism

Forbidden foods
Pork, (including sausages, bacon, ham and gammon), white flour, white sugar, oranges, lemons, grapefruit, tomatoes, vinegar, mayonnaise, rhubarb, butter, cream and spices.
Reduce your daily intake of tea and coffee. Use salt very sparingly; better still, use Dr Vogel's Herbamare in its place.

Recommended foods
Plenty of raw and cooked vegetables, a salad every day, fruit, nuts, honey, cottage cheese, brown rice and yogurt.

Use of herbal and mineral therapy
1. Each evening scald one tablespoon of kidney tea with a pint of boiling water in an earthenware pot or jug (do not use aluminium). The following day drink one cupful to which you have added ten drops of Imperthritica.
2. Take two Alfavena tablets (which are very rich in potassium) and one Kelpasan tablet (which contains Pacific seaweed) before meals three times daily.
3. Take 1,000 2,000 mg of natural Vitamin C each day.
4. Make sure you are not constipated.

My wife suffers from arthritis in her big toes. She has had X-rays and one toe is really bad, while the other is slightly less affected. The only option the doctors have suggested is an operation. Have you any suggestions for this problem?
To my way of thinking an operation is always only ever the last and final resort. Try alternatives first. There are many other ways. For further advice read my book *Arthritis, Rheumatism and Psoriasis.*

My mother's left foot is swollen from arthritis. She is taking codliver oil but wants to know if there is anything else she can take to bring the swelling down?
A swollen foot is a miserable thing because it restricts all movement. The codliver oil is good, but she should also follow my dietary instructions as well as taking a nightly footbath containing bicarbonate of soda.

For years I have had arthritis in the neck and spine. Three months ago my doctor put me on a herbal weight-control programme and within two weeks the pain had gone. Why did this happen and what is in the programme to get rid of the pain?

Probably the diet had a positive influence and the herbal remedies would have helped to relieve pain.

My brother has rheumatoid arthritis. He has had acupuncture and has listened to relaxation tapes. He now feels better but the swellings are still there. Why is this, as he feels so much better?

Relaxation is very helpful and soothing for the body. Visualisation is also of great benefit and will positively influence the condition. However, a good diet and some herbal or homoeopathic remedies may help to speed up the recovery by reducing the inflammation in the joints.

My sister's husband has been taking *Propolis* for his stiff joints. What are your thoughts about this supplement?

Propolis, which is a derivative of royal jelly, is a marvellous remedy for many complaints and a number of arthritis patients have told me how they have benefited from its use.

I have been taking green-lipped mussel extract for arthritis and would like to hear your views on this.

I am very much in favour of this remedy because most people have reported excellent results. For your interest, my book *Life Without Arthritis – The Maori Way* is based completely on this remedy.

While playing with my dog I pulled my shoulder. I now feel as if arthritis has set in and would like to know what to take to prevent this taking a further hold?

Arthritis is often caused by a trauma, i.e. a fall, knock or other injury. When this happens and a swelling appears, take immediate action. Follow an acid-free diet and a good programme such as Dr Vogel's Detox Box Programme.

I am 59 years old and crippled with arthritis. I have been told that I also have Sjögren's syndrome, connected with this.

I take three kinds of medicine for my eyes, but there is no relief. My surgeon now wants to sew up the tear ducts, but I want to know if I could obtain any help from homoeopathic remedies?

This is a sad story and I sympathise with you. Firstly, look for treatment for the cause of your arthritis. Sjögren's syndrome is, fortunately, a fairly rare auto-immune disease which causes dry eyes, a dry mouth, painful joints, and sometimes also respiratory infections.

Certainly homoeopathic and herbal remedies can help, but in view of the severity of your condition please make an appointment with a homoeopathic or alternative practitioner in order to discuss the best course of treatment.

My grandmother is remarkably healthy for her age – 87 years old. At Christmas her knee gave way and she is now in great pain. She has been told that it is arthritis. Can you help?

For a period of three weeks she should place a cabbage leaf poultice on her knee every night before going to bed and leave this in place until the morning. When removing the leaf in the morning rub the joint with Po-Ho ointment.

I have been diagnosed as having psoriatic arthritis in my feet and hands. Specially made shoes have, fortunately, made walking easier, but I would like some advice on diet and exercise.

Several therapies will ease your problems: reflexology, aromatherapy and/or acupuncture. Follow the advice given in my book *Arthritis, Rheumatism and Psoriasis.*

What exactly is osteoarthritis?

Osteoarthritis is a skeletal and muscular condition thought to be primarily caused by ageing. It is also often considered to be a form of menopausal syndrome, triggered by endocrine disturbances, or a traumatic degenerative joint disease. It can indeed be very painful, especially when hard bony swellings have formed.

I am 48 years old and have osteoarthritis in the joints of my big toes. What are the chances of this spreading to other areas?

The early arthritic symptoms are often first detected in toe and finger joints. Take immediate action to try and undo the damage. Usually a balanced diet and Dr Vogel's Detox Box Programme is a good start.

I am 65 years old and have been prescribed zyloric acid. For the last three or four years I have suffered from gout and suspect that this is brought on by alcohol and shellfish. I do not want to be on drugs for the rest of my life.
Zyloric acid is always prescribed for gout. As a rule gout is brought on by rich food, alcohol and acid rich products. Apart from making changes to your diet you can obtain great relief from the remedy Imperthritica, as well as from homoeopuncture, reflexology or aromatherapy.

For some time now I have been having gold injections for rheumatoid arthritis. Whenever I am given more than 20 mg I react very strongly and have now been told to stop the treatment.
In your case I would definitely suggest trying alternative therapies. See a homoeopath or naturopath for more detailed instructions.

I would like to know if aloe vera juice is helpful for arthritis? I am worried because I have been told that it can be dangerous to drink.
I am not aware of any side-effects to aloe vera. Remember, however, that it is also very helpful to use aloe vera cream for rubbing into the joints and this may put your mind at rest.

Recently I had a pain in my hand and it went black like a bruise. This has now cleared up, but the doctor said that it was a form of arthritis. Could this possibly be due to the fact that I have taken *Propolis* tablets for a long time?
I don't think that this can be ascribed to taking *Propolis*. It sounds more like a deficiency of vitamin C. Take at least 2,000 mg per day.

My neighbour is 72 years old and has had arthritis for 30 years. She has had a hip replacement operation to get her out of a wheelchair. She does not eat oranges or lemons because she believes they cause acidity. Neither does she take coffee or chocolate. However, she takes Complan every night, which

is rich in vitamins. Do you think that this helps?

Indeed, Complan is good, but it is not sufficient. Tell your neighbour that she should also take extra calcium, selenium and zinc. Further advice can be found in my book *Arthritis, Rheumatism and Psoriasis*.

I suffer from rheumatoid arthritis in my hands and arms (all my joints). I also have Raynaud's disease, which affects my hands and feet. What is your recommendation?

Firstly you need treatment for your circulatory system. Follow Dr Vogel's Detox Box Programme. Then, for 15 days, take twice daily two 500 IU capsules of vitamin E and 15 drops of Venosan in a little water. Next, for 30 days, take 15 drops of Imperthritica in a little water, together with four Urticalcin tablets, both twice daily.

What are your thoughts on hydrogen peroxide treatment for arthritis?

It is essential that this treatment is only undertaken under the guidance of a qualified practitioner, because it can be harmful when administered incorrectly. It is better to use hydrogen peroxide only for a gargle, and never stronger than 1.5 per cent.

I take my neighbour's black labrador for a walk twice a day, but the vet has advised that the dog should be given less exercise because of its arthritis.

Give the dog a Seatone capsule twice a day and add a spoonful of codliver oil to its food. Continue to exercise him.

Two years ago my husband had polymialgia rheumatica and it was treated with steroids. Now it is returning and we wonder if it can be treated without the use of steroids?

Polymialgia rheumatica is an inflammatory condition affecting the connective tissue in and around the muscles. It mostly affects the shoulders and pelvic areas, causing pain, stiffness and tenderness. Details of alternative treatment methods can be found in my book *Arthritis, Rheumatism and Psoriasis*.

I have had polymyalgia rheumatica for three years and take 5 mg cortisone daily. What would you suggest as an alternative?

Also take three 500 mg capsules of Oil of Evening Primrose daily before going to bed at night and take one GS500 capsule twice daily.

I follow a diet for osteoarthritis. I would like to know what you would recommend as an anti-inflammatory remedy?
Twice daily before meals take 15 drops of Imperthritica and twice daily after meals take 15 drops of *Harpagophytum*.

To aid the treatment of rheumatism, what proportion of codliver oil to Oil of Evening Primrose do you recommend?
Take one tablespoon of codliver oil and three 500 mg capsules of Oil of Evening Primrose before going to bed.

Please tell me what can be taken for arthritis in the thumb (the joints are swollen)?
Twice daily take 15 drops of Imperthritica in a little water before a meal, and also twice daily four Urticalcin tablets.

I have arthritis of the spine. Sometimes when I make a sudden turn or twist I pass out for a few minutes. What causes this?
This is a definite sign that you need manipulative treatment of the neck. Please find yourself a good osteopath and ask him or her for advice.

I am very fond of fruit, but I have heard that it is bad for arthritis. Is this true?
This is not totally true. Most fruits can be eaten without any detrimental effects, with the exception of citrus fruits and unripe tomatoes.

For 50 years I have suffered from osteoarthritis in the knees and for 20 years I have had osteoporosis in the spine. I am 69 years old and, fortunately, I can still walk. I use no medication, but wonder if you can give me advice on how to help the pain?
You have been very lucky so far in that you are still able to walk. Try to improve your condition with a combination of Seatone tablets and Imperthritica drops, which should be of great help.

My wife has a painful right hip and her legs go cold and numb. Is there any homoeopathic cure?

She should take one 500 IU vitamin E capsule twice a day, and Alchemilla Complex will help to relieve the pain and cold feeling.

Is there any hope for degenerative arthritis?
Yes, there is no need to grin and bear it. Seek the advice of a good herbalist or naturopath, and you may also find it useful to read the more detailed advice contained in my book *Arthritis, Rheumatism and Psoriasis*.

I have arthritis in both hands. What should I do when I cannot move the fingers out of their twisted position?
In such cases I have found that homoeopuncture therapy is very often beneficial.

Is it possible to have arthritis pains in the head and could arthritis also affect the eyes?
Yes, arthritis pains can occur anywhere in the body, even in the eyes, tongue and jaws.

Could severe pain in my hand and finger joints be from arthritis?
Usually such pains are due to either arthritis or rheumatism.

What remedy would you suggest for psoriatic arthritis which has steadily deteriorated over the last seven years?
First of all start with a good balanced diet, bearing in mind the dietary instructions mentioned on page 25. In addition, use homoeopathic and herbal remedies and seek acupuncture treatment.

Is it possible for bone that has been damaged through arthritis to grow back again?
It is often amazing how well the body heals. It is not unheard of for bones to lose their swelling and deformities.

What kind of exercise (combined with diet) is best for a mild arthritic condition?
Swimming, walking and cycling are all excellent exercises. None of them is too severe and all are beneficial to overall health.

Two years ago I was to have my kneecap removed. Instead, I

followed your diet for arthritis and I can now walk ten miles at a time. I take green-lipped mussel extract, multivitamins and a mineral supplement. Do you think that I can now stop taking the mussel extract? Can you advise me which vitamins are best for my condition?

Continue with the diet as well as you can, because you have proved that it is effective. The remedies you take cannot do any harm and, again, you seem to thrive on them. For a good multivitamin preparation I can strongly recommend Health Insurance Plus.

When arthritic pains recede should all herbal remedies, pills, etc. be stopped, i.e. Imperthritica, green-lipped mussel extract, Chien Pu Wan and Evening PrimroseOil? If you advise that I have a break from these remedies, for how long should this be?

Always keep taking the remedies for at least an extra 2–3 months after the pain starts to recede. Basically, your body should be able to cope on its own, without their help, because the body heals itself with the help and encouragement of these remedies. Give your body a chance, and if you think that some extra help is needed every now and then, you'll know how to give it that help.

I am 41 years old and have had rheumatoid arthritis for three years. It began in my hands, wrists and feet and has now spread throughout my body. I have been prescribed various conventional medicines, including gold injections, which did nothing to help my condition. For a year now I have been attending a homoeopathic consultant, but the disease continues to progress. How long should I persevere with homoeopathy?

I have no doubt that homoeopathic treatment will be beneficial, but you need patience. You might be able to speed up any improvement with acupuncture, homoeopuncture and additional herbal remedies.

I would be grateful for your advice on the occasional pain I have in both hands, especially my thumb joints. They are becoming a bit disfigured. At the moment I take one aspirin tablet twice a day.

These pains are the early warning signs. Take the necessary steps: adopt a well-balanced diet; take up regular exercise, such as swimming, cycling or walking and use homoeopathic and herbal remedies.

Is it safe to continue taking Seatone (mussel extract) tablets for osteoarthritis?

Yes, this is considered to be a healthy food supplement which is of great benefit for arthritic conditions. Many of my patients have praised this remedy.

What dosage of green-lipped mussel extract do you recommend for osteoarthritis?

Take one capsule before meals three times a day.

My ankle gives way, especially in the mornings, and my right foot tends to swell up. Would reflexology help? Is it alright to take a Kloref tablet – 500 mg effervescent potassium chloride – a day?

Reflexology and aromatherapy certainly help conditions such as yours. As to your second question, potassium is nearly always deficient in arthritic people and this remedy can therefore only be to your benefit.

Several of my friends, out of pain and desperation, are ordering 'cure-all' books and pills, touted to be arthritis cures etc., from mail order advertisements. What is your general opinion of this type of product?

I must warn you that my personal feelings on this subject are very negative. It is difficult to judge, but I would be careful with any commercially marketed panacea. I would much rather see that your friends consult a qualified practitioner who can help and guide them with knowledgeable advice.

My mother has very painful wrists due to over-use and a touch of arthritis. They are swollen. The doctor suggests painkillers, which my mother does not like taking on an ongoing basis. Do you have any advice on diet or homoeopathic remedies? My father is diabetic and my mother follows the same diet he takes.

Certain joints that are often used may become stiff and sore and they will need a bit of extra help. Even though your mother follows a healthy diet, she will probably benefit from herbal remedies such as Imperthritica and Alchemilla Complex.

There was a medical man from America on the television and radio some weeks ago who recommended taking a tablespoon of codliver oil in two tablespoons of milk in the morning on an empty stomach as a remedy for rheumatism and arthritis. I have taken this for 6–8 weeks and it seems to be helping, but now I am concerned that so much codliver oil may somehow be harmful. I also control my arthritis by diet and since having had allergy tests I have cut out dairy products.
I have heard some encouraging reactions to this therapy, but would not advise this to be taken on a long term basis. The body needs a variety of foods, and overdosing in any shape or form is always unwise. Consult a doctor or a naturopath, who can keep an eye on your condition.

What is lupus erythematosus?
This is an auto-immune disease that causes inflammation of the connective tissue, in particular the membranes of the joints.

Having recently been told that I have a type of rheumatic disorder called SLE (systemic lupus erythematosus), I am keen to see a naturopathic practitioner. I would like to see if an alternative treatment is available for my condition. How do I go about seeing someone such as yourself?
Always make sure that the person is qualified and registered with a bona fide organisation. You may like to ask the Health Practitioners' Association or the Homoeopathic Medical Association for a recommendation.

If your bones continually crack does this mean you will be arthritic when you are older? Is it true that this could just be a family tendency?
This is often a sign of the onset of osteoporosis.

Would there be unfavourable side-effects from using Vogel's detoxification course for a long period of time (as opposed to once or twice a year)?

I doubt that there would be any detrimental effects, but this excellent cleansing programme is not required more than once or twice a year.

Can anything be done to help relieve pain in the legs caused by a lack of blood to the nerves due to spinal stenosis?

Take one 500 IU vitamin E capsule twice a day and use the herbal remedy Venosan 15 drops twice daily.

What are the possible causes of arthritis?

Arthritis can be caused by infections, allergies, a hereditary tendency or inflammation. However, arthritis can also be triggered by trauma, e.g. jealousy, an unhappy marriage, unemployment, resentment, etc.

I suffer from systemic lupus erythematosus. I have what has been diagnosed as a cold sore, which appears on my cheek whenever I get an attack. Have you any suggestions or comments?

Always take 2 g of vitamin C daily and take 15 drops of *Harpagophytum* twice daily.

What advice could you give for osteoarthritis of the cervical spine?

Soft-tissue massage and acupuncture, combined with herbal remedies will bring much relief.

Is there a specific diet for arthritis?

Yes, but the diet is dependent upon the exact type of arthritis. More detailed recommendations are given in my book *Arthritis, Rheumatism and Psoriasis*.

Once osteoporosis has been diagnosed and fractures sustained, how can one ensure that further demineralisation of the bone does not take place, bearing in mind that calcium and vitamin D, if taken, are not necessarily absorbed where required by the bones. Can any form of complementary medicine help?

Osteoporosis can be helped by following a balanced acid/alkaline diet. Bone deterioration can happen after a certain age, but it can also be greatly reduced by the use of a calcium supplement that is easily absorbed, such as Dr Vogel's Urticalcin or Osteo Balance from Nature's Best.

What are your suggestions for hip pain in a 60-year-old. My X-rays are clear and I am currently taking non-steroid anti-inflammatory drugs. Severe pains induce nausea, which frequently wakes me up. Some days are better than others.
Take 15 drops of Imperthritica in a little water twice daily. Drink herbal teas and follow an acid-free diet.

Are painful shin bones a sign of anything specific?
People are often surprised to hear that this symptom is usually caused by tension.

I have had ankylosing spondylitis for about 16 years. Can the damage be undone and will it affect my children?
Ankylosing spondylitis is an auto-immune disease where the joints become inflamed, before stiffening and finally fusing together, causing the spine to lose its suppleness and become rigid. It has a strong tendency to run in families. Although such damage cannot be reversed, many patients who have been treated with acupunctue have managed to keep the condition under control. Acupuncture will help, as will the use of Symphytum officinalis, Seatone and codliver oil.

Is there anything in particular that can ease the pain of arthritic knees?
Acupuncture will help and also herbal remedies.

If a person keeps to a strict low-acid diet to combat arthritis is there not a risk of affecting the effective digestion of food by not having enough acid (i.e. hydrochloric acid) for this purpose – thus giving rise to other problems?
Our intake of acid is usually higher than we realise. It is extremely unusual that your fears become reality, and if that were the case the situation could quickly be adjusted.

What exactly is scleroderma and what homoeopathic treatment would you recommend as opposed to steroids?
This is a rare auto-immune disease where the smallest blood vessels and capillaries become inflamed, after which they shrink and harden. Try to avoid exposing yourself to excessive heat and consult a qualified homoeopath for individual advice.

What causes loss of cartilage and what can one eat to restore it?
Take five Urticalcin tablets and also 15 drops of Symphytum officinalis twice daily. Both remedies will be of great benefit.

My husband has scoliosis of the spine. Are there any exercises to help this condition, e.g. yoga?
Yes indeed, yoga may well help. However, any of the exercises described in my book *Neck and Back Problems* will be beneficial. An example of a simple but useful exercise is to stand erect with the back, heels and head all against a door and try to slide the back up and down, keeping the body pressed flat against the door all the time. He may prefer to place a chair in front for support. Eventually, he will have enough confidence to do the exercise without the chair.

My friend had a fall on the coccyx and she has experienced pain in the lumbar spine ever since. She was diagnosed as having osteoarthritis in the lumbar spine and curvature of the upper spine. She also suffers badly from asthma. What is your advice? She is also upset as she has been referred to a psychiatrist as this is obviously not seen as a physical problem.
The coccyx is a very tender part of the spine and ends in three little crystals that are easily damaged and mentally the pain can affect a person badly. This, together with her asthma can easily cause depressive bouts. Personally, I doubt the value of seeing a psychiatrist. Please suggest that she consult a good acupuncturist or osteopath. Sometimes some gentle manipulative adjustment of the coccyx can relieve the pain.

My mother has spondylitis. It started with a slipped disc seven years ago. She now walks bent over and cannot straighten herself up. She is in constant pain. The hospital has just discharged her saying that there is nothing more they can do for her. She is on eight painkillers a day.
Please try homoeopuncture!

When I do neck exercises I hear a grating sound. I am not in pain, but wonder if these exercises could be harmful?
If you would rather not stop your exercise classes, take great care with

these neck exercises. Often this signals the beginning of arthritis and you should treat these symptoms as a warning.

My neck and left hand are very painful. I used to play squash, but had to stop because of the pain. I have had physiotherapy for eight months where they 'stretched' my neck which relieved the discomfort. But tiredness and stress bring on the pain again. I have stopped the physiotherapy because I was told they could do no more for me.
Usually where physiotherapy fails, osteopathy succeeds. To combat your tiredness and stress take *Ginkgo biloba* tablets, which are also good for the blood circulation.

I wonder if you could recommend a remedy for stiffness in sports people? I am an enthusiastic golfer, but am becoming progressively stiffer.
For all sports people I would suggest the use of selenium, calcium and zinc as mineral supplements. Garlic and Oil of Evening Primrose capsules can also be helpful.

My husband is 50 years old and for the last couple of years he has had 'housemaid's knee'. Life is a misery for him. He has been to a bone specialist and has had acupuncture – all to no avail. What is the answer?
'Housemaid's knee' can indeed be a misery, but it can also be relieved quite quickly with homoeopuncture. An old, but effective, remedy is to wrap a cabbage leaf around the knee at night. Also try rubbing the affected joint with PoHo ointment daily.

I have had considerable back trouble which was diagnosed as spondylitis. Then I heard about green-lipped mussel extract and am now on my second bottle. I am not sure if it is my imagination, but I am already feeling better. Is this possible?
I have prescribed this remedy for the best part of twenty years now and most of my patients have thrived on it. This is one reason why I wrote a book about this wonderful remedy, *Life without Arthritis – The Maori Way*.

Is there anything I can take for fibromyalgia?
Because it can be such a painful affliction I would advise the following:

1. Homoeopuncture.
2. Imperthritica – fifteen drops, twice daily.
3. Oil of Evening Primrose – three 500 IU capsules before going to bed.
4. Soft-tissue manipulation.

My wife suffers from both cervical spondylosis and 'trigger finger'. Can you suggest a treatment for either complaint?
Homoeopuncture is the most suitable form of treatment. This is a combination of homoeopathy and acupuncture and the treatment is usually performed by qualified acupuncturists. She should also take two 500 IU vitamin E capsules daily.

My mother-in-law has Paget's disease and she suffers a great deal of pain. We would like to know if there is a homoeopathic cure?
To relieve the pain she would be best advised to undergo acupuncture treatment. I would also suggest that you read my book *Arthritis, Rheumatism and Psoriasis* for details of further therapies she could try.

Is there a cure for stiffness in the hip joints?
Rheumatism and arthritis often starts with stiffness in the joints. Start treatment immediately: the programme should include a healthy and balanced diet, codliver oil, Imperarthritica and garlic capsules.

When an X-ray shows osteoporosis is there a natural way to replace the lacking hormones, and if so, what is the remedy?
Yes, natural substitutes for HRT (hormone replacement therapy) are available. I would, however, suggest that you seek the guidance of a qualified naturopath for a personally designed programme.

Is there an alternative to HRT for the treatment or prevention of osteoporosis?
Take, twice daily, five tablets of Urticalcin, which is a calcium preparation that is relatively easily absorbed by the body.

Is there anything that would alleviate the pain of osteoarthritis in the knees?
My recommendation is to try acupuncture treatment. Also, on alternative

nights, place a cabbage leaf on the knee and use a bandage to keep it in place overnight. In the morning rub the knees with Symphytum.

How can I reduce arthritic swellings of the finger joints?

Take 2g of vitamin C daily, 15 drops of Imperthritica in a little water twice a day, and at night three 500 mg capsules of Oil of Evening Primrose.

Is there anything I can do to stop a recurring rheumatic pain (in my neck or shoulder)? The pain goes after taking Voltarol.

Voltarol is a painkiller and therefore I would suggest that you should try to treat the cause of your problems instead of the symptoms. For further advice read my book *Arthritis, Rheumatism and Psoriasis* and follow the programme referred to as Dr Vogel's Detox Box Programme.

For three years I have had pain in the back of my legs – above and below the knees. What can I do?

Each day, take two 500 IU vitamin E capsules, Symphytum, selenium and three 500 mg capsules of Oil of Evening Primrose.

My sister-in-law is 41 years old and is married with three children. For years she has suffered from muscular rheumatism. She is unable to take anti-inflammatory medication due to a stomach ulcer. Please can you give her any help and advice?

Advise her to follow a programme made up of the following:

1. A healthy and balanced diet.
2. Water treatment (hydrotherapy)
3. Codliver oil.
4. Imperthritica.

Following an American's advice I take one tablespoon of codliver oil per day on an empty stomach for osteoarthritis. I do not, however, follow his advice regarding drinking only ten minutes before eating, and never with or after a meal. Is this advice really necessary for the oil to be beneficial?

It is always good to take remedies a little before or after meals. The digestive system needs a little breathing space.

Do you think there is any connection between arthritis and the additives and chemicals that are added to beef?
Certainly! Many cases of arthritis are caused by such offenders. Arthritis and rheumatism are blood diseases and waste and toxic matter are often the cause.

My mother would like to know if taking Aloe vera juice is helpful for arthritis. Someone has told her that it can be dangerous to drink this juice.
To my knowledge it is not known that Aloe vera has medical side effects, but tell your mother that it is also helpful to use Aloe vera cream for rubbing onto the joints.

I would like to know if there is any alternative medicine for arthritis of the spine?
Seek acupuncture treatment and use herbal teas, seatone, Symphytum, Imperthritica and garlic capsules.

What general treatment would you advise for rheumatic aches and pains?
Read the answers to the other questions in this section. The overall treatment for rheumatism and arthritis is fairly similar. As with arthritis, rheumatism patients are advised to follow an acid-free diet. Any muscular pains and cramps may be early warning signs of rheumatoid arthritis.

I have rheumatic pains in both knees and am in considerable pain and discomfort. Can you recommend any homoeopathic treatment or remedies?
Pay attention to the dietary guidelines for rheumatism and arthritis. Take 15 drops of Imperthritica twice daily and, where possible, seek electro-acupuncture treatment. A very old remedy, yet a most effective one, is to fold a cabbage leaf over the affected joint before going to bed at night, keeping it in place with a light bandage. In the morning rub the joint with PoHo ointment Keep using a cabbage leaf poultice for several weeks at least; the PoHo ointment may be used for an unlimited period.

What can you recommend for osteoarthritis in the hips?
I usually prefer to give my patients with osteoarthritis in the hips acupuncture treatment. I would also recommend Seatone and codliver oil.

I have rheumatic pains in both my shoulders and feet. My doctor has told me that I have too much calcium in the blood. My main problem is that I cannot walk very well and wonder if you could give me some dietary advice?

First of all I would refer you to the dietary guidelines. Furthermore, I should also explain the fish oil theory, because a fish oil supplement would be advisable for your condition. The fish oil theory generated fresh interest in the 1980s, when Eskimos were found to have lower levels of LDL cholesterol and higher levels of HDL cholesterol than the Danes. In particular, fatty acids in the fish oil consumed by Eskimos are thought to be the reason why the Eskimos can eat such a high-fat diet and yet maintain a healthy heart.

The special and beneficial ingredients in fish oil are two unusual Omega-3 fatty acids, EPA (eicosapentaenoic acid) and DHA (docosahexaenoic acid). The first of these is known to be a crucial component in the body's production of prostaglandins (hormones), concerned with metabolism and manipulative enzymes. We cannot readily obtain these fatty acids from any other dietary source and sometimes the body's own synthesis of them from other dietary fatty acids is inefficient, so a supplement source can be useful.

Cold-water, oily fish such as herring and mackerel are rich in EPA and DHA and yet the more popular fish consumed, such as cod, haddock and plaice, are poor providers of these fatty acids. The Omega-3 fatty acids are thought to be much more effective than the Omega-6 ones in keeping the blood thin and the circulation moving – even in extremely cold environments. They are indispensable for the formation of healthy cell membranes and help to maintain normal levels of fat in the blood. Frying or the prolonged boiling of fish removes the beneficial oils from the flesh.

I have very bad osteoarthritis and would like to know which oils to take and how much? I have heard about codliver oil cures, but would like your opinion.

Read the answer to the previous question for information on fish oils. You may also like to try Seatone, which is an extract of the green-lipped mussel, imported from New Zealand. This has provided tremendous relief from rheumatic pains for many people.

I have been on a diet for arthritis for two years now – no red meat, citrus fruits, alcohol or sugar – as I was supposed to

have my kneecap replaced. So far I have been able to get by
without this surgery. I also take green-lipped mussel extract
every day.

You seem to have done very well so far. If you get the opportunity I would
also recommend electro-acupunture treatment as part of your
programme. Keep up the good work!

**I have heard you mention treatment for rheumatic aches in
the ankles. Could you please repeat them for me?**

Rub the ankles with Symphytum every day and, if possible, undergo
some acupuncture treatment.

How beneficial is green-lipped mussel extract for back pain?

I have seen many good results in my patients who took Seatone. Please
read my book *Life without Arthritis – The Maori Way* for more details about
this remedy.

**I would be interested to learn if anything can be taken for
epilepsy and rheumatism?**

For both diseases a number of herbal or homoeopathic remedies may be
used. I would suggest that you read my books on the subjects. However,
at the same time I would like to warn you that Oil of Evening Primrose
should *not* be taken by people with an epileptic condition.

**I have a son aged 29 who has recently been diagnosed as
having rheumatism in one of his hips. He has been given a
type of cortisone injection, which has not really helped a
great deal. Have you any suggestions?**

Considering the young age of your son I must stress that action should be
taken immediately. The programme I would be most likely to recommend
for him would include acupuncture, Seatone in combination with fish oils,
Imperarthritica and, if possible, some physiotherapy.

**Could you please let me know if there is a remedy for
inflammation of the joints due to rheumatoid arthritis?**

Take one Seatone capsule three times daily and follow the general dietary
guidelines provided on page 26.

ASTHMA AND BRONCHITIS

Why is it that cases of asthma and bronchitis seem to be so much more common nowadays?
I believe the main culprits to be a lack of balance in the diet, too much dairy produce and air pollution.

Could you please explain to me the difference between asthma and bronchitis?
In short, asthma is a partial reversible obstruction of the major and minor airways of the lungs due to inflammation and contraction of the muscles in their walls.

Bronchitis is an inflammation of the mucous membrane lining of the airways in the lungs, and this condition can either be acute or chronic. In my book *Asthma and Bronchitis* I have explained about many of the difficult breathing problems that are prevalent today.

Two years ago I noticed that I was beginning to get breathless and my lungs would wheeze on exertion. After trial and error my doctor gave me a mild steroid inhaler which is keeping the problem under control, but I may have to use it for life. My age is 56 and I would be pleased to hear your advice. Last year I also developed high blood pressure and I am now on tablets.
For both problems, the breathlessness and the high blood pressure, you need help from a qualified medical practitioner. Remember that a naturopath or homoeopath may be able to advise you on possible alternatives to steroids.

I suffer from asthma and for some reason the symptoms become worse in July and August, when I have to increase the use of my inhaler. The problem is that periodically I lose my voice for no reason at all. Specialists say that there is nothing wrong. I sing in a choir and can sing one day and then not the next, because I have lost my voice. I have tried steam inhalations but they brought about no noticeable change. Can you advise me?

Do not worry too much because I have successfully treated patients with similar complaints. I have found that gargling with Molkosan helps and, oddly enough, a supplementary iron intake also helps. Try taking Iron 24 mg Amino Acid Chelate from Nature's Best.

My neighbour's little boy is five months old. They are a family of chronic eczema and asthma sufferers. They have refused to have their son immunised and have consequently been struck off the doctor's list. Can you suggest anything?

Everyone ought to be registered with a practitioner and you might like to point out to your neighbours that they could register with a homoeopathic or naturopathic practitioner, who will guide them. Very often, eczema and asthma are interlinked because of an allergy to dairy foods.

I am 52 years of age and four years ago I developed asthma. I now seem to get colds all the time. What can I take to prevent these colds?

It seems to me as if the immune system needs some help. Always bear in mind that prevention is better than cure. I would suggest that you take 20 drops of Echinaforce and one Imuno-Strength tablet twice daily and 2 g of vitamin C daily.

I have had chronic bronchitis for four years. How can I get well?

A positive attitude will help you to turn the corner. Read my book *Asthma and Bronchitis* for further advice and you will be surprised how many self-help methods are available.

Could you recommend a basic treatment for chronic bronchial asthma, and also tell me how to build up the immune system?

For your bronchial asthma I would advise the following programme:

1. Follow a healthy and balanced dairy-free diet.
2. Seek individual advice on homoeopathic or herbal treatments.
3. Take regular, but not strenuous exercise.
4. Practice Hara breathing exercises (see my book *Stress and Nervous Disorders*).

To build up the immune system I would suggest that you supplement your diet with Nature's Best Imuno-Strength.

As an asthma patient I have been on steroids for many years. Is there any way that I can safely reduce my intake?
The only way to reduce a dependency on steroids is under careful medical guidance, and this always must be done very, very slowly. From experience I can assure you that it can be done and any practitioner will be happy to help you cut down your steroid intake.

If a 13-year-old asthmatic child were taken off his medication (Pulmicort inhaler daily, Phyllocontin tablets, and Ventolin when required), would alternative medicine be able to help him?
As explained above, I would advise you to go ahead with this only under strict medical supervision and even then very gradually. Too many patients have made the mistake of discontinuing long-term treatment in an ill-advised manner and have suffered because of it.

Years of bronchial problems have damaged my lungs – the doctors say permanently. Their medical advice was to learn to live with my condition! I find it difficult to accept this and wonder if there is an alternative in homoeopathy? I am female and in my fifties.
Certainly the body can heal itself if we set it on the right course. There are plenty of ways to encourage this healing process: diet, natural remedies, breathing exercises, etc. Read my book *Asthma and Bronchitis* for further details.

I suffer from asthmatic attacks after exertion. What advice can you give me?
Be careful not to exert yourself, because nothing is gained by it. Read up on what is available as a relaxation therapy and select the programme or therapy that most appeals to you and would best fit in with your life style.

I have very bad asthma. Please can you tell me what I can do to help myself to get better?
Follow the dietary guidelines in my book *Asthma and Bronchitis*. Take

remedies such as ASM drops, Echinaforce, Usneasan, garlic capsules, and practise breathing exercises.

Are all asthma sufferers, both adults and children, allergic to milk?

Although many asthma patients are allergic to milk, this is not always the case. Most are allergic to some substance or another, however, and other traumatic influences are also relevant.

Have you heard of treating asthma by owning a cocker spaniel?

No, I have never heard of any such claim and I would be extremely suspicious of any such suggestion. On the contrary, it is a well-known fact that many allergies are actually caused by domestic pets.

How can I help children who use inhalers for asthma? I take them for yoga classes.

Inhalers are usually designed for quick relief. When considering a change over to complementary natural remedies that actually treat the cause of the problem, it should be remembered that this can only be achieved very gradually and must be done under strict medical guidance.

What treatment do you recommend for bronchitis? I have continual phlegm in the chest and even when walking I get breathless.

1. Drink herbal teas.
2. Reduce your intake of dairy foods.
3. Twice daily, take 20 drops of Echinaforce before meals.
4. Twice daily, take 20 drops of Bronchosan after meals.
5. Take three garlic capsules before going to bed.

I have just purchased your book *Asthma and Bronchitis*. Do you mention how to treat bronchial pneumonia with remedies? If not, what are the best remedies? I do not have TB, but was told in the USA that I have the TB germ and given the right circumstances I would be prone to TB.

Bronchial pneumonia is described in Chapter 3 of the above-mentioned book. The diagnosis reached in the United States obviously referred to a

TB miasma, which is a leftover from a previous inflammation, infection or virus, and which will certainly make you more prone to the actual condition. Take good care of yourself and it may not come to anything.

My friend's three-year-old son was recently diagnosed as suffering from asthma. Can you offer any advice?

Young children with asthma are often allergic to dairy foods, although this is not always the case. The allergy may be to a different substance. Ask a homoeopathic or naturopathic practitioner for individual advice.

Over the last year or so I have developed a wheeziness. Asthma does run in the family, unfortunately.

Do not forget that asthma or asthmatic conditions can be the result of an allergy. Arrange for tests to determine the cause and take the appropriate action.

What is your recommended treatment for chronic bronchitis?

Chronic bronchitis can be a very unpleasant condition. An effective treatment programme should include dietary measures and remedies, such as ASM drops, Bronchosan, and Oil of Evening Primrose. Seek the advice of a medical practitioner.

How would you treat someone who suffers from asthma (due to house/dust mite)? I am also frequently bothered with rhinitis attacks.

First of all you should be tested for allergies, after which a homoeopathic nosode can be decided upon for dust or house mite, if indeed that is the cause of the allergic condition. Also, use the remedies *Harpagophytum* and ASM drops and take garlic, either fresh or in capsules.

I visited your clinic a few years ago, but today's question is for my granddaughter, who is aged two. At the moment she is suffering from an asthma attack, which began three days ago, and six months ago she suffered a similar attack. The doctor gave her Ventolin. I wonder if she could be allergic to dairy produce? The little girl loves milk and my daughter will not deprive her of it unless she is sure that this is the offending substance.

I cannot say for certain that she is allergic to dairy produce, but I would not be surprised. Why not try her on goat's milk or soya milk instead of cow's milk?

B

BACK AND NECK PROBLEMS

I have back and neck problems and friends have suggested that I consult an osteopath. However, I do not know much about osteopathy.

Osteopathy is a system of medicine which places the chief emphasis on the relationship between structural integrity and health. The body is endowed with the means of sustaining optimum health but this can be impaired by mechanical defects. Gross defects usually come within the category of orthopaedic lesions, whilst the osteopathic lesion may, in itself, be very minor and difficult to detect. Frequently, such lesions are nothing more than loss of joint tolerance, which may give rise to joint pain and limitation of movement.

Although osteopathy is most often used for musculo-skeletal problems, it is also employed effectively for other disorders and it is well established that manipulation of the spine can alter neuro-endocrine and neuro-visceral activity and thus affect general health. Osteopaths traditionally regard the vascular system as being of prime importance and employ a fair amount of soft-tissue manipulation.

Can you please give me some general advice on how to overcome and avoid back pain?

Back pain can have different causes and unless I am given specific details of your symptoms I could talk for hours without even coming close to mentioning your specific condition. I would suggest that you read my book *Neck and Back Problems*.

I am registered disabled and have pain directly on the lower spine. On occasions the pain moves to either side and up the spine. I have also received treatment for coeliac disease, but

unfortunately without success. I have now been told to go home and use the painkillers that I have been prescribed. There is no more to be done. Can you tell me if there is anything that I can do to reduce the pain?

My recommendation is acupuncture treatment. Also, for external treatment try rubbing the spine with Symphytum and take internally 15 drops of Imperarthritica and two capsules of Seatone twice daily.

My husband is suffering from a ruptured disc in the back. He has had traction and heat treatment, to no avail.

Every day he should take a hot, leisurely bath to which a handful of bicarbonate of soda has been added. Acupuncture treatment also often brings relief. Twice a day he should take 15 drops of Alchemilla Complex before meals, together with four Urticalcin tablets.

I go to an exercise class and when I do neck exercises there's a sound like bone grating on bone. It does not hurt, but even so I wonder if I should stop exercising?

Do not stop exercising, but make sure that the exercises you do are gentle ones. It is good to keep the neck mobile and therefore gentle exercising is necessary. I can understand that the grating noise causes you concern and I suggest that you take Alchemilla Complex together with Urticalcin.

I have a herniated disc which causes back pain. Is there any cure?

You should consult a qualified practitioner who will probably give you homoeopuncture treatment. This is a combination of homoeopathy and acupuncture. Also, take 20 drops of Alchemilla Complex twice daily.

My husband suffers from tendonitis and cortisone injections have not worked. He is now seeing a chiropractitioner, although so far this also does not seem to be working. Do you think he should continue to attend this clinic?

Sometimes tendonitis takes time to recover. Personally, as well as manipulation I also give my patients acupuncture treatment. I also advise them to rub the affected area with some warm olive oil.

I suffer from a tennis elbow and would like to know if there is an alternative treatment to cortisone injections?

From the large number of tennis and golf elbows I have treated, at a conservative guess I would say that at least half of these patients had had cortisone treatment before coming to my clinic. Both golf and tennis elbows can be effectively treated by manipulation and/or acupuncture and/or laser treatment. It may come as a surprise to learn that the majority of the sufferers appeared to have a shortage of zinc. Therefore I often prescribe a zinc and copper supplement.

I have a prolapsed disc. Some specialists suggest I have surgery, while others recommend physiotherapy and an exercise programme. What do you think?
You are possibly describing the prolapse of the intervertebral disc, and if that is the case, surgery is not always needed. Bear in mind that once the disc has been removed it can never be replaced. See a qualified osteopath, chiropractitioner or acupuncturist first before making up your mind about surgery. Also, read my book *Neck and Back Problems* for further suggestions on treatment methods.

My friend is in her seventies and has a weak bladder and suffers from slight incontinence. She takes peppermint medicine for a hiatus hernia and receives nerve medication for spondylitis of the spine. When she walks even for only a short distance she gets very tired, and yet she can play the piano for three hours at a time without any problem. She has also started breaking out in cold sweats. Can you help?
Firstly, the weak bladder may be a result of the spinal problems. Every disc or vertebrae has a function to all the organs of the body. Obbekjaer's Peppermint is good for the digestive system, Cystoforce from Dr Vogel will help the bladder and the cold sweats may be helped by *Salvia*. However, I would suggest that your friend see a naturopath or osteopath for advice that is specifically designed for her condition.

Eighteen months ago I had a slipped disc and was given physiotherapy in hospital. Usually I slept on the floor, but once I laid down on the settee and couldn't get up. The only way to get off the settee was to allow myself to "fall" off. This damaged my leg and I was taken to hospital where I was given an epidural, which deadened the lower part of my body. I was told that it was sometimes successful and

sometimes not. Part of my leg still feels dead. Can you suggest something?

An epidural is not always necessary. In my practice over the years I have treated numerous similar cases and still do. Oesteopathic treatment usually solves the problem, and sometimes acupuncture or massage is also applied. The dead feeling in your leg can soon be overcome by taking supplementary vitamin E and, twice daily, 20 drops of Venosan.

I apparently injured a cervical disc in a car accident and have been told that it has developed into a C6/C7 nerve root infringement. What should I do now?

Be wary of manipulation and remember that soft-tissue work and patience may be helpful. Find a qualified practitioner because I do not doubt that Curapulse or Diapulse treatment may well help your problem. Clinical and experimental studies conducted in the past 35 years show that many of the effects of high frequency energy are due to electromagnetic effects other than heat. Diapulse therapy was developed to take advantage of this important finding and to increase the range of applications of this valuable new form of treatment. It has been shown to be of special advantage as an adjunctive therapy in accelerating the normal process of bone and tissue healing, as well as in the treatment of osteomyelitis, bursitis and rheumatoid arthritis. Diapulse can be used safely with patients of all ages, with no danger of tissue damage due to overheating. It can be used effectively through clothing, plaster casts and surgical dressings, and over metal implants. There have been no reported contra-indications to the use of Diapulse in over three decades of clinical application.

My husband suffers from sciatica, which affects his job as he does a lot of driving. Tablets such as distalgesics do not have much effect. What can he try?

There are relatively few real cases of sciatica. If indeed a person does suffer from sciatica the pain can be excruciating. Often, sciatica is caused by a spasm of the piriformas muscle, which is found in the buttocks. If the piriformas muscle goes into spasm it causes pressure and the sciatic nerve which runs underneath causes the pain associated with sciatica. I usually treat such a condition successfully with homoeopuncture and a few natural remedies. Your husband may benefit from reading my book *Back and Neck Problems*.

I recently had an X-ray which showed that the disc spaces in my spine were narrowing. The discs are pressing on the nerves, causing my knees and legs to ache. I am now having acupuncture, but I wonder if this is the best remedy or can you suggest anything else?

Narrowing or compression of the discs can be very painful. Already you have started with acupuncture, which is good. But as the protection of the disc has become worn or degenerated, I suggest that you also take some remedies to try and reverse the damage, e.g. Imperthritica, Symphytum Urticalcin, zinc and selenium.

My husband has a trapped nerve in his neck, which gives him headaches and means that he cannot sleep at night. He has tried acupuncture and reflexology, which haven't worked. What is your recommendation?

A neck condition such as your husband's often causes considerable problems. I usually give acupuncture treatment and soft-tissue manipulation. Sometimes, when the resulting restriction of the blood supply is causing dizziness, I also suggest the use of herbal remedies such as Venosan or Aesculus Hipp.

My husband is 57 years of age and generally in good health. For five weeks now he has had bad headaches and has been given pills for trapped nerves. They have not done any good. What would you suggest?

Headaches are alarm signals indicating that something somewhere is not right. If the pills for trapped nerves have not helped your husband then the headaches are likely to be caused by another reason. This shows how damaging an incorrect diagnosis can be, because the time lost before receiving the correct treatment can hinder and delay recovery. Swallowing pills or painkillers is easily done, but this is creating a nation of chronic invalids. Suggest to your husband that he seeks the advice of an osteopath or chiropractor.

My sister sprained her ankle seven years ago and the bit of leg above the ankle bone is still a little swollen. Is there anything she can do to get rid of the swelling?

Seven years is an awfully long time for a swelling to remain. It is possible that some bone in the foot is out of place and from experience I would say that this is usually the cuboid bone. Your sister may want to seek a second opinion. I would also suggest that she rub *Arnica* ointment onto the area.

My husband has suffered from aching legs from the hips down for a number of years now. He has had X-rays and there appears to be no sign of arthritis in his hips. He is a printer by trade and therefore has to stand for much of his time at work. Is there anything you can suggest to relieve the aching as it is getting worse?
In many such cases simply taking supplementary vitamin E will help (500 IU, twice a day).

I have a condition of the lumbar spine, described as follows: degenerative bone changes in LV3, LV4 and LV5, with sclerotic bone changes in LV4 and LV5 and narrowing of the LV3 to LV4 and LV4 to LV5 disc spaces. What should I do?
In the first place make sure that you have a well-balanced and healthy diet. I would further suggest that you seek acupuncture or manipulative treatment. Also use some remedies, such as Alchemilla Complex, Urticalcin or Osteo-Balance.

I have been suffering from a frozen shoulder for over a year now and have had both NHS and private treatment, but have not found any relief. Cortisone treatment has been recommended but because of the side-effects I am not keen. Will the shoulder cure itself or should I have cortisone injections, or have you any other suggestions?
A frozen shoulder can indeed be a sore affliction and I have seen patients fainting with the pain. Over the years I have found that the best results are obtained with acupuncture, homoeopathic injections and gentle rubbing with warm olive oil. Take 15 drops of Imperthritica twice daily. A helpful and gentle exercise is to place a rolled up bath towel in the armpit and gently press the arm against the body.

Five months ago I broke my wrist. I had a Colles' fracture and some broken nerves. The hospital said that it will never fully recover, but the physiotherapist says that if I work at it, it may improve, although it could take as long as a year. Is there anything I can do to help the nerve situation?

Although physiotherapy is very worthwhile I have found that the best results can be obtained with acupuncture and laser therapy. Also, take some herbal remedies, such as *Galeopsis* and Urticalcin.

What is your advice for the treatment of tendonitis?

Tendonitis can be greatly helped with acupuncture and acupressure treatment. Seek a qualified practitioner who will advise you.

I have suffered from back trouble for the past 38 years. Now I have been offered the chance of a spinal operation which has a fifty-fifty chance of success. I cannot decide whether to go ahead or not.

It is near enough impossible for me to advise you unless I can examine your back. My best advice must be that you first consult a qualified osteopath or chiropractitioner. Surgery must always be the very last option, when all else has failed.

How can I help myself? I suffer from low back pain and neck pain which causes migraines. I know that I suffer from a lot of tension, which does not help my complaints.

Back and neck pains can be very persistent and draining. You must get help. It may well be that your migraines originate from a neck condition, but they could also be caused elsewhere. Find a qualified osteopath or naturopath and explain your condition.

What is the treatment for inflamed nerves, especially due to a herniated disc?

Take 15 drops of Imperthritica and some Folic Acid twice a day.

What can be done for calcium accumulation in the shoulders?

Do some gentle exercises and twice daily take ten drops of Petasan after meals.

What treatment would you recommend for inflammation of the elbow?

At least once a day place the elbow in a basin of warm water in which a teaspoon of bicarbonate of soda has been dissolved.

My leg muscles are wasted because of polio and the condition is deteriorating. Can this process be slowed down? Maybe I should also mention that at night I have burning hot feet.
Acupuncture treatment will help and I would suggest that you also take a vitamin B complex supplement.

I have had a stiff shoulder for the past four or five months. How best should I treat this?
Keep it warm and rub it daily with warm olive oil. Where possible, massage and manipulation are also advised.

What are the possible causes of muscle spasms in the side of the neck?
It is most likely that sudden muscle spasms are caused by either tension or an awkward movement. Do some gentle exercises and read up on relaxation techniques.

Is yoga an appropriate treatment method for a damaged disc in the lower back? It seems to have helped to ease the pain down my leg. Will yoga be sufficient on its own to heal the disc, if it can be healed at all?
One should always be careful with exercises and I must warn you not to overdo things. A new aerobics class in the area of our clinic always brought about a spate of new patients. Any form of exercise should be gentle and comfortable. Yoga in itself will not heal a disc, but for this purpose you may use Oil of Evening Primrose capsules and the homoeopathic remedy Symphytum.

I have had a sore back now for at least six months. Is it possible to treat a compressed disc? My doctor has told me not to have any other form of treatment other than what he suggests.
I can neither agree nor disagree with your doctor because I do not know what treatment he has suggested for you. I will add that for conditions of a compressed disc I have seen some very good results achieved by acupuncture.

What is the best remedy or treatment for a prolapsed disc between the shoulders and the neck?

Each morning and night take 25 drops of Alchemilla Complex together with four Urticalcin tablets.

My friend broke her spine and had a laminectomy and bone graft operation. However, she still gets cramp, from her hip right down into her foot. Can you advise her?

The cramp could possibly be due to muscle and nerve pressure. Tell your friend to take some gentle exercise, e.g. walking, swimming and cycling. She may also be advised to take two 500 IU capsules of vitamin E daily.

Can you tell me if there is a herbal medicine to counteract the pain of bursitis?

Bursitis is an inflammation of the little pads (bursea) around the joints and tendons. Acupuncture treatment will help and I would also suggest that you rub the affected area daily with some Po-Ho ointment.

I am 25 years of age and a professional football player. I find that any injury I sustain takes much longer to correct itself than previously. Can anything be done to speed up the healing process?

By continuing to play, rather than rest, after you have sustained an injury, the constant movement this entails means that it is bound to take longer to recover. It will, however, help if you take *Arnica 3x* twice a day and also three capsules of Oil of Evening Primrose last thing at night.

I have a calcified piece of bone and a steroid injection did not help. Is there anything else I could do to help as it causes me a lot of pain?

I have helped many people with cold-fire frequency treatment. Laser treatment will also be beneficial, as will rubbing the affected area with Symphytum ointment.

My husband has suffered from acute back trouble for many years. His doctors can find neither cause nor cure. Today he is in extreme pain after having sneezed earlier. When this happens it causes pain to travel up his spine which leaves him near enough crippled for a while. Could you tell us the cause and how best to cope with this? We would also appreciate some advice on possible remedies.

In many cases such an acute condition is caused by a weakness in the muscles and ligaments. Believe me when I say that it is certainly not in the mind, as some people may suggest. I feel that acupuncture and/or manipulation treatment would be best, with the addition of a vitamin B complex, zinc and a calcium supplement.

A student in my class complains of dizziness when bending forward (she does not suffer from high blood pressure, but has a history of giddiness and fainting). She also complains of neck pain. I thought all this may be caused by tension, as she is a working mother. Do you have any suggestions?
I am tempted to agree that stress and tension may be at the root of the problem. This can cause a restriction in the blood supply to the brain, causing giddiness and fainting. Please advise her to visit an osteopath or naturopathic practitioner.

Since I attended a Shiatsu seminar I have had lower back pains. My doctor suggested that this is due to muscle spasms, but after seven weeks there has been no improvement. I still have not been able to rejoin my yoga classes. Have you any suggestions?
Sometimes unusual exertion or exercise can bring on muscular spasms and if this has been going on for seven weeks I feel that some manipulative treatment may be needed. Seek the advice of an osteopath or chiropractitioner.

What would you do for a neck whip-lash injury of a few years' standing?
A whip-lash injury must never be under-estimated as it can lead to unsuspected symptoms, such as losing the hair or nails. A whip-lash is a serious condition and must be treated under medical supervision. Remember that much can be done with alternative medical treatment, and tissue-healing is also important. My suggestions would be acupuncture treatment, soft-tissue manipulation, laser treatment and herbal remedies.

My daughter is 14 years old (and according to X-rays is no longer growing) and has major lumbar and thoracic scoliosis with a rib hump. Is there anything that could help her

straighten her spine? I do not want her to have surgery (spinal fusion). Does having your ears pierced damage you (e.g. by losing a piece of your ear that may be an acupuncture point)?

Acupuncture certainly will help your daughter as well as exercises. You are correct in your latter assumption, because ear-piercing can indeed go right through an acupuncture point. It never does to interfere with the energy balance in the body. For more detailed information on this topic, please read my book *Body Energy*.

What can be done, if anything, for my dear daughter-in-law after one year and nine months of conventional hospital treatment for whip-lash caused by a road accident (leaving her with pain in her neck, shoulders, arms, back and face)?

Without doubt she can be helped by acupuncture treatment, laser treatment and remedies such as Alchemilla Complex and Urticalcin.

My friend has psoriatic atrophy and is receiving gold injections, which do not seem to be helping. She suffers from labyrinthitis and all her joints are affected, especially the spine. Can you help?

If all else has failed, why not try alternative treatment? I am convinced that homoeopuncture and herbal remedies will help. Tell your friend to seek the help of a qualified acupuncturist or homoeopathic practitioner.

I have a tingling sensation in my left hand and feel that this may be caused by some damage I sustained to my elbow several months ago.

Very likely you are correct in your self-diagnosis. Make sure that the elbow is treated and for this purpose I would suggest Curapulse or Diapulse treatment. Also, take 15 drops of Venosan twice a day.

The problem is a trapped sciatic nerve in the hip. Apart from having had osteopathic manipulative treatment (most effective so far) I have also had vitamin injections and painkillers. However, the problem is recurring. Traction and plaster-cast treatment have also been tried. If the answer is vitamins, which vitamins should be taken?

I feel that homoeopuncture may be the answer, together with some Folic Acid and Vitamin B100 Complex from Nature's Best.

My husband has back and neck pain which travels to his arms and elbows. The doctor prescribed a liniment, but it hasn't helped. He is 53 years of age and there is a history of arthritis in his family. Can you tell me if there are any homoeopathic cures that may help him?

There are a number of homoeopathic remedies that could be used, but in all fairness every practitioner would prefer to see the patient and decide on his own diagnosis. In all cases I would suggest *Arnica*, but please try and persuade your husband to make an appointment with a homoeopathic practitioner.

I have calcification of an old muscle tear in my knee. When it became inflamed my doctor prescribed anti-inflammatory drugs (Brufen) which have a very irritating effect on my stomach. Is there a natural method of preventing the condition from flaring up and, better still, of curing it? I have recently taken up yoga, but my knee is preventing me from doing all the exercises.

As you quite rightly mentioned, Brufen is an anti-inflammatory drug and I would suggest that you try instead Dr Vogel's remedy Imperthritica. Also, rub the knee with PoHo oil.

BLADDER WEAKNESS AND BEDWETTING

My six-year-old daughter is devastated that she still wets the bed. How can I help her?

For some strange reason, especially for girls, the homoeopathic remedy *Pulsatilla* is very helpful in such cases. For external treatment laser therapy is very good. Bedwettting in boys usually requires a different approach. I would advise taking ten drops of Cystoforce twice daily. Neither boys nor girls should be allowed to drink after 5.00 p.m. Before the child goes to bed rub St John's Wort Oil over the region of the bladder and between the legs. Alternatively, try the remedies *Sabal* or *Solidago*.

I am 78 and suffer from recurring cystitis. Can you please tell me how herbal medicine could be of help for my condition?

For your complaint I would definitely suggest that you use Cystoforce, as herbal remedies can be of great help. Herbalism is a naturopathic treatment method. Apart from the fact that herbal medicines are of entirely natural origin, in naturopathic treatment the diagnosis and treatment relate to the individual rather than to a specific disease. Allopathic treatment may consist of a single drug for a specific condition, but herbal treatment will work mildly and gently to rebalance the body, ensuring that there are no toxic side-effects. There is an energy inside every human body which science is unable to quantify or explain. Herbalists call it the 'vital force' which inspires the body to life and their approach to health is chiefly concerned with maintaining its equilibrium. If this delicate balance is encouraged, it means the whole person enjoys good health. If it is disturbed the result is disease. Herbalism aims to treat the patient, not the disease, by directing the vital force and encouraging it with herbal remedies which stimulate the body's own defences to produce the desired return to positive health.

For some time now I have had bladder problems. I have taken the homoeopathic remedy *Sepia* for an irritable bladder. Is there anything else you could recommend that may be more effective? I have already used Oxybulynin, but this affected my eye muscles and therefore I was advised to change to *Sepia*.
Although *Sepia* can be used, I am more inclined to prescribe *Pulsatilla* and Cystoforce.

Would you be able to give me some advice for my grandson, who is nine years old and still wets the bed regularly?
Give the boy ten drops of Cystoforce twice daily and rub St John's Wort Oil over the bladder area and between the legs before he goes to bed. Make sure he takes no liquid after 5.00 p.m.

I need to pass water very often. Although I do not eat after 4.00 p.m. and never drink after 3.00 p.m., I am still up frequently during the night. What would you advise?
Without a doubt your bladder is weak and needs some attention. I would suggest acupuncture or laser therapy. Cystoforce is also very good for strengthening the bladder, and you should remember to use salt sparingly.

Could you please advise me on how to treat a bladder infection?

Use the natural antibiotic Echinaforce daily until the infection has completely cleared.

What is the best way to overcome frequently recurring attacks of cystitis?

As above, use Echinaforce daily.

How would you treat chronic bladder infections and urinary tract pain?

Three times a day, take 15 drops of Echinaforce before meals, and twice a day, take ten drops of Petaforce after meals.

Do you have any advice on a suitable diet for chronic cystitis sufferers? Can you also recommend any herbal remedies to help cystitis?

Use salt very sparingly and eat plenty of celery and Celeriac. Take 15 drops of Cystoforce twice daily.

I am being treated for urinary incontinence. I am 53 years old and have a history of torn ankle ligaments, a slipped disc and torn rib muscles. What can I do or eat to cure my incontinence.

Your incontinence should be treated with Cystoforce, a zinc supplement and D complex vitamins. For your other problems take Alchemilla Complex (20 drops twice daily).

I am 36 years old and struggle with problems of urinary frequency and urgency. I also have thrush on the tongue each morning and irregular bowel movements. Do you have any suggestions?

To relieve the need to pass water frequently take 15 drops of Prostasan twice daily and every day eat a handful of pumpkin seeds. Thrush can often be cleared with Molkosan: twice a day, take a teaspoonful in half a cup of water. To regulate your bowel movements chew half a teaspoon of Linoforce granules twice daily.

BLOOD PRESSURE

What can be done about high blood pressure?

First of all, the underlying cause of this condition must be discovered and in this your practitioner will be able to help, although you may have to undergo several kinds of tests. Once the cause has been diagnosed, the appropriate action can be taken. This action may consist of any one or several of the following indications:

1. A well-balanced diet with little or no salt.
2. Relaxation exercises.
3. Herbal or homoeopathic remedies.
4. Possible temporary use of drugs if the blood pressure is very high.

Our circulatory system works like a central heating system. If the pressure is too high, a weak point in the pipes may expand and eventually burst. The last thing we want is for an artery to sustain such damage and therefore it is very important that immediate action is taken. You will find much useful advice in my book *Heart and Blood Circulatory Problems.*

It appears to be much less common than high blood pressure, but how serious is low blood pressure?

Unfortunately, low blood pressure is equally as bad as high blood pressure. The same advice applies as above: find the cause. This can be something as simple as tiredness or an iron deficiency, but it could also be more serious. Sometimes vitamin E (500 IU twice daily) and the herbal remedy Hyssop will help. Also, dietary management will be beneficial: eat plenty of beetroot, carrots, spinach, green vegetables and alfalfa.

Can anything be taken for low blood pressure? I have had two brain operations and wonder if this may have any relevance to my low blood pressure?

You will be perfectly safe to take one Hyssop tincture twice daily.

What can you recommend for an 82-year-old person who suffers from high blood pressure and constipation?

Constipation is a problem for many people, but especially so for people with high blood pressure. Remember that whatever is imported into the body should be exported within the space of 24 hours. Twice a day, chew slowly one teaspoon of Linoforce. You may find that once the constipation has been overcome, the blood pressure may also normalise.

For some time I have suffered from high blood pressure and dizziness. How does homoeopathy work?

The dizziness can be greatly helped by taking three Arterioforce capsules daily.

As to your question on homoeopathy, ever since Dr Samuel Hahnemann formulated his system based on the principle 'Like Cures Like', it became a complete medical treatment. Hahnemann became dissatisfied with the explanations for the action of allopathic drugs and decided to examine their effect on perfectly healthy people. He tried the drug *Cinchona* on himself, and was amazed to discover that it produced in him the very symptoms of the diseases which it was supposed to cure. He repeated the experiment, using different drugs on other volunteers, and his findings led to the reiteration of the great healing principle once pronounced by Paracelsus: *Similia Similibus Curentur.*

Remedies diluted one part in one hundred more than thirty times over became commonplace in homoeopathic prescribing, which led to ridicule from allopathic doctors and 'conventional' scientists, who, quite rightly, claimed that none of the original substance could possibly remain. Homoeopaths were not so ignorant as to be unaware of this, but they held that a healing force was unlocked when a substance was succussed and diluted. In short, homoeopathy treats people, not the disease.

What can I do about angina, pains in my hands (swollen knuckles) and aches in both feet?

Please read my book *Heart and Blood Circulatory Problems* and carefully follow the dietary instructions.

Does ginseng help in cases of high blood pressure?

No, I would hesitate in prescribing this for my patients. I would be more likely to select the remedy Ginsavena, which is a composition containing ginseng and *Avena sativa.*

What are your views on hypertension and your recommendations for treatment?

In my books *Heart and Blood Circulatory Problems* and *Stress and Nervous*

Disorders you will find detailed information on this subject. It is likely that you will be able to borrow these books from your local library.

What is the natural treatment for hypertension and circulation problems, and I also wonder if you have advice for overcoming impotence?

For hypertension and circulation problems I would suggest the following programme:

1. Dietary management.
2. Relaxation therapies.
3. Herbal remedies.

Because of your hypertension you need to be aware of certain remedies which are marketed for the specific purpose of counteracting impotence and therefore I would strongly suggest that you discuss this with your doctor or practitioner.

I have high blood pressure and also suffer frequently from stomach upsets which cause bouts of vomiting. Can you give me some advice?

It is possible that you have been prescribed drugs to balance your blood pressure and that you react unfavourably to them. Take ten drops of *Centaurium* before meals three times daily.

What kind of treatment do you advise for high blood pressure?

First and foremost I advise my patients on a suitable diet. I would therefore suggest that you consider trying the rice diet outlined in my book *Heart and Blood Circulatory Problems*. Also, take Arterioforce capsules and fresh garlic or garlic capsules.

I have too much iron in my blood. Can a change of diet help?

Most certainly. To follow a diet with a lower iron content is most definitely the best advice I could give you.

Do you have any thoughts on why men are more likely to suffer from heart disease than women?

I am not sure whether this is correct or not, but most people appear to ascribe it to the fact that men tend to undergo more stress at work. Equally important factors, however, are that on average men smoke and drink more. Obesity also plays a part. It should be noted, however, that recent years have seen an increase in the number of women affected by heart disease.

About 25 years ago I had a heart attack. I am still taking what is called 'the water tablet'. Can I cut it out, because my ankles are no longer swollen?

In all fairness to your practitioner, you ought to discuss this with him or her. He or she may agree to reduce your tablet intake slowly, or even better, may advise you to take a herbal remedy in its place.

What advice for maintaining good health would you give to a young person with a ventricular septal defect?

First of all, ensure that you have a healthy and balanced diet. I would also suggest the use of *Crataegus* (five drops after meals, twice daily).

Can you explain why I should experience a heart flutter on waking up in the morning? All night this is in my subconscious and really worrying me. I am 33 years of age and work as a sewing machinist – a pressurised job.

This problem could be due to stress induced by your work. You would be well advised to ask your doctor to check your blood pressure. I would also recommend that you take *Crataegus* (five drops after meals, twice daily).

What can I do for calcification in my mitral valve, which appears not to close completely? I have an irregular heartbeat for which the doctor has prescribed medicine to thin the blood.

You ought to continue taking the medication prescribed by your doctor, but at the same time you could take five drops of Petaforce after meals.

My sister suffers from dropping or low blood pressure, especially when she stands for any length of time. Her doctor has no solution.

Suggest to your sister that she tries to do some light exercises and also takes twice daily five drops of *Crataegus* after meals.

According to information in *The Swiss Nature Doctor* by Dr A. Vogel, raw carrot juice increases the blood pressure. Do you agree?

Yes, but only if taken in large quantities. This is the reason why people with low blood pressure are advised to drink this regularly. However, the blood pressure is not affected when carrot juice is taken in moderation, e.g. half a glass daily.

I need to know what I can do to control my blood pressure in a natural manner. I have never taken any medication, but I have been told that for the last seven or eight years my blood pressure has been too high. Recently it has gone higher than ever before.

Read my book *Heart and Blood Circulatory Problems* for dietary advice. In particular, you should eat three times a week some brown rice prepared in the manner described in this book as part of the dietary recommendations.

I have read that vitamin E is good for high blood pressure. Is it safe to be taken by someone with mild angina?

Always be very careful. I have seen patients taking 1,000 IU of vitamin E daily who developed tachycardia. If you want to take vitamin E, never take more than 200 IU twice daily.

C

CANCER

Can cancer be cured?
The word 'cure' is a very big word in relation to cancer, but I have seen many patients who had achieved a large measure of 'control' for their condition.

What do you think of the 'Moerman diet' for cancer?
Recently this dietary programme has been thoroughly tested in the Netherlands and the eventual prognosis was very positive.

I would be interested to learn your opinion of the 'Iscador' treatment for cancer patients.
Under good medical supervision the Iscador or *Viscum album* (mistletoe) treatment has helped many cancer patients. For more details please read my book *Cancer and Leukaemia*.

Twice I have undergone surgery for breast cancer and yet it has recurred for a third time. I have now been told that, meantime, it has spread to the liver and bones. My doctor has suggested chemotherapy, but I am afraid.
Follow your doctor's advice and complement this with a good diet, extra vitamins, minerals and trace elements and some herbal remedies.

I am 48 years old and have six-monthly check-ups for cancer because my mother died of breast cancer at the age of 54. I take Evening Primrose Oil and codliver oil daily, which have been recommended by the doctor. However, he advised me not to take HRT although I am going through the menopause and am plagued by symptoms of hormonal imbalance.

In your case I wholeheartedly agree with your doctor's advice and would leave HRT (hormone replacement therapy) well alone. Continue with his programme and also make sure you have a balanced diet. You could also use supplementary vitamins and Petaforce.

What do you think of the 'Gerson' anti-cancer diet (intensive juices, vegetables, no meat, little animal protein, no fats, coffee enemas, etc.) which seeks to replace sodium in the diet with potassium?

The Gerson diet has been of tremendous help for many people. I have seen many very ill cancer patients returning from the Gerson clinic in a much improved condition. You can read all about the Gerson therapy in my book *Cancer and Leukaemia*.

As a tumour and cancer treatment is there value in the Canadian herbal combination called 'Essiac', that has powdered sheep sorrell as the basis?

In Canada I have met a number of patients who had taken Essiac, with a varying measure of success. To my knowledge this remedy is not available in Britain.

Why do calm, well-balanced, well-fed people get cancer? It appears to be a contradiction in terms?

Many kinds of cancer nowadays are thought to be caused by stress and tension. However, cancer still is a mystery in many ways and to my way of thinking it depends entirely on the influence and effectiveness of the immune system.

My friend suffers from chronic leukaemia and has a viral infection. Both conditions are affecting the glands in her neck, which have become very swollen. Her doctor has told her that there is no treatment for her condition. Is there anything you can suggest?

First of all one should always remain positive. If need be, use a visualisation technique to encourage positive thinking. You must never stop trying. The other day I saw a patient who was told 20 years ago that she only had one month to live. She is still with us and this could well be because she took positive action at the time and decided to help herself! You may like to read up on these aspects in my book *Cancer and Leukaemia*.

Do you have any theory on bone cancer? I know someone who was recently diagnosed as suffering from bone cancer and as the cancer has spread so far the only advice was hormonal treatment. Are there any homoeopathic remedies?
Tell your friend to consult a homoeopathic practitioner for individual advice. This should be done without delay.

Some two years ago I wrote to you about alternative medicine and received a very encouraging reply. I would like you to know that I have continued to stay well since, leading a busy and normal life. It is almost three years since I had surgery for breast cancer. I take my vitamins regularly, but I also think that attitude is one of the greatest things in helping this condition. I take the very greatest pleasure in being able to send you my sincere greetings.
This lady was prescribed a dietary regime and supplementary vitamins to help boost her immune system. To my mind the functioning of the immune system lies at the root of good health or ill health.

I have heard of diets for diabetes, ulcers, kidneys, etc. I would like to know if there are any special diets for cancer sufferers?
You will find an example of a well-balanced diet for cancer sufferers on pages 113–114 of my book *Cancer and Leukaemia*.

I am a great believer in the saying 'Prevention is better than cure'. For a person who has just started a six-month chemotherapy programme for the treatment of Hodgkin's Disease, would you have any suggestions, e.g. to continue and re-evaluate my nutritional requirements, to alter and correct the problem?
Alongside your chemotherapy treatment make a determined effort to follow a good nutritional programme. With chemotherapy and radiotherapy one must never forget that as well as killing off the bad cells, some good cells are also destroyed. Cell renewal is necessary for life. Therefore you should aim to use vitamins, diet and natural remedies to boost the immune system.

My son has had leukaemia for two and a half years. The chemotherapy has affected his liver and he may have to go

back into hospital for liver treatment. Is there anything in the homoeopathic field that could help to improve the condition of his liver?

You will find some specific advice if you read my book *Cancer and Leukaemia*. Liver cleansing may also be beneficial, and the Vogel remedy Boldocynara always aids the liver function and encourages it to perform its tasks more effectively.

Is there anything you can recommend to help women with breast cancer? It may be diet or treatment. I would also like to know what women can do who have recovered from breast cancer, and as a preventative measure.

A healthy life style is, of course, always of the utmost importance in any case of illness or disease. Take care of your diet and ensure that you have sufficient relaxation. Take supplementary vitamin and mineral preparations and recognise the important role of the immune system.

What is the name of your book on the subject of cancer?

My book is called *Cancer and Leukaemia* and is available from most good book stores and healthfood stores, or in local libraries. In this book you can read about many aspects of cancer and find out about the advantages and disadvantages of varying alternative therapies.

Last January I had a lymphoma in the face and had radium treatment for a month. Is there anything I can take to help my condition?

Yes, by all means. Make sure that you use a full spectrum of vitamin supplements and also Oil of Evening Primrose.

I very much enjoyed reading your book *Cancer and Leukaemia* and when my husband was undergoing radiotherapy for an astrocytoma brain tumour we used an alternative approach. He also has seizures, is 27 years old and awaiting his results.

For the seizures he may find the herbal remedy *Loranthus* helpful. I am touched by your letter and hope that the advice you have found in my book will be of long-term benefit to your husband.

How do you feel about using Tamoxophan for preventing the recurrence of breast cancer?

The drug Tamoxophan is often prescribed after surgery. Your doctor will advise you when it is time to reduce or stop the intake of this medication. Then you will have to take it into your own hands to try and rebuild your immune system. I would suggest that this is the time to start taking 2 g of vitamin C daily.

With your vast experience have you come across any laboratory type of work involved in cancer research? Do we have any faint hope?
In Paris there is a laboratory where orthodox and alternative medical researchers work closely together. Hopefully, this co-operation will become more common, as both branches of medicine are essential and dedicated to reduce human suffering. In articles on the subject I have read that in the USA and Mexico there are similar research laboratories where this close co-operation takes place.

Medical doctors have told me that the cancer I had could be cured with chemotherapy, but if it did come back, they then could do no more than control it. What should one do to reduce the chances of cancer coming back?
In all circumstances one should follow a healthy diet, and never more so than in a case such as yours. You should also take vitamin C, herbal remedies, and ensure that you have sufficient rest and relaxation.

CANDIDA ALBICANS

Can you tell me briefly what a *Candida albicans* condition is?
Candida albicans is a yeast parasite that lives in all of us, but in some people it is active and in others it is non-active. More detailed information can be found in my book *Viruses, Allergies and the Immune System*.

What are the foods to avoid for Candida?
In cases of an active *Candida albicans* condition one should not eat or drink any fermented products (yeast-based), mushrooms, sugar, chocolate, wine or cheese.

At present I use Tyne-Lotrim to cure my recurrent yeast infection. How can I cure the cause in a natural way? Why do I keep getting yeast infections?

The best way to keep a yeast infection under control is by remembering to avoid the above-mentioned foods. There certainly are conventional medicines such as Caprylic Acid and Nystatin, that can be used but also herbal remedies such as *Harpagophytum* and *Spilanthes* have proved very effective. *Biodophilus* and *Acidophilus* will help to avoid the infection becoming active.

In someone suffering badly from *Candida* would *Candida 30* be a better homoeopathic treatment than the *Smillimum*?
Yes, because many times I have seen a remarkable improvement when *Candida 30* was used.

I am recovering from a combination of Candida and hypothyroid – Hashimote's thyroiditis – that severely undermined my immune system. The last couple of years I have followed a wholefood diet and used vitamin and mineral supplements (extra vitamins C and E), supplementary juicing and a thyroid supplement. Is this correct or do you have any better suggestions?
It is very sensible to help the immune system with additional vitamins and minerals. A food supplement specifically designed for just such conditions is Imuno-Strength, and also the herbal remedy Nasturtium is often of great help.

Please could you tell us some more about the treatment of candidiasis and its relation to food allergies, especially in which cases you would advise the use of Echinaforce?
Echinaforce is an extremely useful and effective natural antibiotic, but also it is a good remedy to help the immune system. One should never underestimate *Candida* problems, and must try to keep this condition under control, and if possible to banish it from the system.

I have a chronic rash on my face. I believe it is due to candidiasis and currently I am on level 1 of the Trowbridge anti-*Candida* diet – and have noticed some improvement in the skin of my face. Can you suggest anything for further improvement?
You are on the right road with the diet you are following, but it may help to speed up your progress if you take 15 drops of *Harpagophytum* twice daily before meals.

How should one take Devil's Claw for *Candida*? Are there any other remedies you would advise for the treatment of *Candida*, and how soon can the problem be cleared up?

Devil's Claw or *Harpagophytum* is certainly an excellent remedy for the treatment of this yeast condition. You may also like to try using Acidophilus Plus, and I would like to explain in some more detail why a healthy diet and digestion are so important for this condition. The digestive system plays a vital part in achieving successful nutrition. It doesn't matter how careful you are at guarding your intake of micronutrients, to achieve optimum nutrition, or even adequate nutrition, your digestive system must stay healthy.

Food taken into the body must first be broken down into molecules small enough to be absorbed. This is done by enzymes, which are protein molecules themselves, that break up large molecules of fat, protein and carbohydrates into smaller pieces, releasing other nutrients at the same time. These nutrients must then be absorbed through often quite complex biochemical processes which transport the nutrient molecules across the gut wall. All this must be achieved while the body strives to maintain a favourable balance of bacteria in the digestive system. Nature's Best has developed a powerful but friendly range of supplements designed to support the natural good health of the digestive system.

The gastro-intestinal (GI) tract of a normal healthy individual plays host to a very large and varied population of micro-organisms. In an adult the total weight of bacteria will amount to approximately one kilogram. In healthy individuals, that microbial population is delicately balanced and only when this balance is maintained does the GI tract function effectively. The quality of the body's intestinal flora is determined by the balance between the various microbial species, especially the two predominant groups, the beneficial bacteria and the putrefactive bacteria. *Acidophilus* species are regarded as beneficial and tend to counterbalance the putrefactive bacteria.

The bacterial balance should remain stable throughout life, although certain factors such as illness, excessive yeast growth, changes in diet, travelling abroad or treatment with antibiotics can upset the balance. Also, it has been shown that in the elderly, the presence of beneficial bacteria is often significantly reduced, which may account for age-related changes in the working of the GI tract.

The principle of helping to sustain a favourable balance of the beneficial bacteria with supplements containing live, viable bacteria has been established for some time now. The supplements have become more and more sophisticated as manufacturers tackle the enormous problem of stability. Even though the bacteria have been freeze-dried they are still alive and they rely on stable conditions to maintain them in a state of suspended animation. Potent live *Acidophilus* products can now be manufactured under very strict conditions, which will help the user to maintain this precious bacterial balance.

I have been diagnosed as having *Candida*. How can I keep the symptoms at bay?
Start immediately, and perhaps the first step should be to follow the internal Detox box Course for 15 days and follow the anti-*Candida* diet instructions which can be found in my book *Viruses, Allergies and the Immune System*. At the same time you could use some remedies such as *Harpagophytum* and Echinaforce.

You have mentioned the remedy Devil's Claw for candidiasis, but are there any other remedies you might like to suggest?
Candidiasis can be a very unpleasant and persistent condition. Low-grade infection with *Candida albicans* can cause all kinds of thrush, vaginal, vulval and penis problems. Yeast, moulds and dietary deficiencies can be the cause. All kinds of problems can occur from such infection, for example headaches, a bloated stomach, diarrhoea and allergies. As well as Devil's Claw you may like to think about using supplementary vitamins A, B and C, zinc, magnesium and *Acidophilus*.

CHOLESTEROL

The doctor tells me that my cholesterol level is too high. It appears that diet can combat this, but what else can be done about it?
Please understand that if you were to get rid of your cholesterol you would be dead! Cholesterol in the body is essential, but the level of cholesterol must be balanced. If your cholesterol level is above 5.2 points, this is a sure sign that some attention is needed. Unfortunately, cholesterol is nowadays a much blamed and misunderstood condition. The gelee forming on the inside wall of the artery does not kill. The loose particles which travel through the artery are dangerous and could possibly result in

a stroke. This lining on the inside of the arteries is usually caused by alcohol, nicotine and too much animal acid. Read my book *Heart and Blood Circulatory Problems* for more detailed information.

I have been warned that my cholesterol level is too high. How do you suggest I get it down?

Follow a fat-free diet and remember, no smoking and no alcohol. Understand that it is better to take very little butter in preference to a poor margarine, but it should only be very little. Eat plenty of fruits and vegetables. Every day eat a handful of grapes, remembering to chew the seeds carefully. Also use oral chelation and take Boldocynara twice daily.

Is it true that hawthorn berries are good for controlling the cholesterol level and do you have any other suggestions?

Yes, you are quite right, and furthermore I would strongly advise the herbal remedy *Vinca minor* (periwinkle extract).

Can you suggest a remedy to counteract hardening of the arteries?

Use FLW tablets – oral chelation therapy – two or three times a day. The principle of oral chelation is explained in more detail in my book *Heart and Blood Circulatory Problems*.

What would you suggest for the treatment of gout and high blood pressure?

Both problems should be tackled immediately. Speak to your doctor and begin without delay taking the appropriate dietary measures as suggested in my book *Heart and Blood Circulatory Problems*.

What are your recommendations in order to lower cholesterol and blood pressure – diet or herbal remedies?

Both! Read the answers to other questions on these topics.

Is there a homoeopathic alternative for the orthodox water tablets (Frusemide)? I have heart problems and fluid on the lungs.

Frusemide is a long-term drug and without permission from your medical practitioner it would be very unwise to discontinue this programme. Ask him or her for advice.

My latest medical check-up revealed a cholesterol level of 10.2. I was told this is high. Is this true?

Yes indeed, a cholesterol reading of 10.2 is very high. Please don't waste any time, but read the relevant chapter in my book *Heart and Blood Circulatory Problems* and take steps to reduce this cholesterol level immediately.

I have a cholesterol problem, and a vegetarian diet together with the drug Probucol have been ineffective. At present I am taking MaxEpa fish oil, but the results are as yet unknown. Can you suggest anything I can do to help overcome the problem?

I would also take two or three oral chelation tablets daily.

For someone trying to reduce her cholesterol level, can you tell me if facial cream absorbed through the skin is detrimental? This may contain a lot of cholesterol.

You need not worry on this score, facial cream will not affect the cholesterol level in the blood. Follow the recommended dietary instructions carefully.

What do you think about Lopid in the treatment of cholesterol? What vitamins can be used to reduce high cholesterol levels?

Vitamins, flax-seed oil and Silymarin are all effective means to reduce the cholesterol level. Please note that Nature's Best will give you free information on the conditions for using these remedies.

CIRCULATION PROBLEMS

What would you suggest for poor blood circulation?

Take plenty of exercise in the fresh air. Exercise need not be strenuous in order to be effective; walking and cycling are ideal. Swimming is another good form of exercise, and one which involves the whole of the body in a gentle way.

A further specific treatment for poor circulation is the hydrotherapy programme, also known as 'cold dip'. This exercise should be done first thing in the morning on rising and each night on retiring. At the side of the bed place a basin of cold water and have a towel ready. On waking up in the morning, place both feet into the water. Having counted to ten, remove your feet from the basin and place them on the towel to damp dry. Exercise your toes as if trying to pick up a marble. Do this 10–30 times. At night, before retiring, follow the same procedure as suggested for the morning. You will find that your feet are glowing and warm when you go to bed. An important thing to remember with this exercise is that it should be done for a minimum of 60 days if you want to feel the benefit. Although this exercise sounds very simple, I can assure you that if carried out correctly, you will benefit greatly.

What would you do for cleansing the blood?

Follow one of the fasting programmes described in my book *Food* in the Nature's Gift series. Drink plenty of herbal teas such as camomile, stinging nettle, golden rod and nasturtium. Also, consider following Dr Vogel's Detox Box Programme.

I have poor circulation which causes chilblains and 'dead fingers'. Is there anything that can be done?

Chilblains can be greatly helped with *Ginkgo biloba*, Hyperisan, Urticalcin and homoeopathic injections. I have often found that enzyme injections, e.g. Vasolastine, are very helpful.

What could the possible cause be for numbness and pain from the elbow to the fingers?

Such a pain could be caused by pressure on the elbow, or pressure on the ulna. This may require osteopathic treatment, but until the cause has been correctly diagnosed it is impossible to give you a more specific answer.

I waken early every morning with cramp in both ankles and legs. This started with one leg, but now both legs are affected.

This sounds very much like a circulatory problem and I would suggest that you read my advice in the rest of this section regarding exercise and dietary measures.

I suffer from severe attacks of cramp and wonder if you can suggest a better cure than magnesium phosphate?

Sometimes Magnesium Orotate, together with additional vitamin E is effective. Nature's Best has a suitable supplement which also contains selenium.

My sister has poor circulation in lower legs and feet, as well as painful ankles (I must admit that she is overweight). She uses a parsley and birch foot balm, and also other herbs to counteract fluid retention. She has a good herb garden and wonders if there are other herbs she could be using?

She cannot go wrong if she used thyme, rosemary, sage and garlic in her cooking. Also St John's wort, stinging nettle and nasturtium can be of great help.

What is Raynaud's disease and is there a suitable homoeopathic remedy for treatment of this disease?

Raynaud's disease is a condition in which there are functional changes in the blood vessels of the fingers and toes. Sometimes other parts of the body are affected as well. Again, the advice is the same as that for improving the general blood circulation: exercise and dietary control.

My mother was an active 84-year-old until last month, when she lost the use of her legs. She also had pins and needles in her fingers. Now her hands feel dead and she cannot hold a cup. The ends of her fingers feel heavy and her hands are very cold. Gradually, she is regaining the use of her legs. The doctor has said that it was not caused by a stroke, and her blood pressure is normal, although she does take soluble aspirin. What do you think is wrong with her and how can I help her to regain the use of her hands?

The symptoms described are not uncommon in elderly people, but they can be due to several causes. The best and safest way to help her would be to give her twice daily the Bioforce remedy Arterioforce (2 capsules).

What would you suggest for severe and recurring cramp in the legs?

Please read the answer to previous questions on this subject. Spasms of leg cramp can be quickly overcome if the foot is placed in cold water, on a cold floor, or on a cold and wet towel. Try stretching the leg, pulling the toes towards the knee.

What can be done about leg ache?

This can be due to a variety of reasons, but mostly you will find that additional vitamins E and C will help. If it persists you should go and see your practitioner.

I have a chronic circulatory problem in my left leg. Also, there is the problem of lymphoedema. Doctors are of the opinion that nothing more can be done. I have been told that if my leg deteriorates there is little chance of saving it. Would you be able to make any suggestions?

It is possible to treat lymphoedema and if you already have consulted doctors, I would therefore suggest that you ask a homoeopathic practitioner for advice. Over the years I have used several herbal remedies, depending upon the circumstances, which have proved effective.

I have always had poor blood circulation. How can I get rid of spider veins below the ankle bones? I have high blood pressure: 180/100 and 160/90.

First of all you must make sure that your blood pressure is treated effectively. For the spider veins I would suggest that you use Venosan, Urticalcin and *Aesculus hipp*.

What causes cramp in a leg in the middle of the night and what can be done about it?

Cramp is often due to the position of the body while asleep. A simple way is to put a cushion under the mattress at the bottom of the bed so that the feet are raised compared to the rest of the body. Also, take extra vitamin E.

Can a chiropractor help to overcome numbness and blanching of the fingers and toes, and what kind of diet would you suggest for this condition?

Sometimes treatment from a chiropractor or osteopath is effective and it is certainly worth trying. As far as diet is concerned, follow the general rules for a low-protein diet.

My niece is 15 years old and she complains that her thighs and legs go numb at night, which stops her from sleeping. Sometimes her wrists go numb during the day. Rubbing them

does little or no good. Her doctor prescribed Feldene, which has had no success. Can you help?

This sounds very much like a disorder of the circulatory system and I would suggest that this is looked into first. Be very careful with the use of sugar and salt and take supplementary calcium. Use the 'cold dip' treatment as described on pages 78-79 and rub the affected areas with St John's Wort Oil. Regular exercise will help to improve the circulation.

What would you suggest for bad circulation of the hands, with the fingers going white, etc.?

In most cases Venosan and *Aesculus hipp.* work well. However, acupuncture treatment and/or massage can also be beneficial.

What actually is phlebitis and is there a natural treatment?

Phlebitis is an inflammation of one or more veins. This is mostly caused by toxicity in the blood. Taking 15 drops of *Hamamelis virg.* (witch hazel) twice daily is often very helpful.

Can you say anything about thrombosis?

The term 'thrombosis' describes the condition where a blood clot forms on the rough and inflamed wall of a vein or an artery. Due to sluggish circulation and high blood-lipid levels, the affected channel may become restricted. Take ten drops of *Hamamelis virg.* (witch hazel) twice daily.

I not only suffer from bad circulation (cold hands and feet), but also from poor short-term memory. What is your advice?

For both problems *Ginkgo biloba* is good, or oral chelation as described in my book *Heart and Blood Circulatory Problems*.

I get numb feelings in my left foot. What can I do to improve my circulation?

This numbness may be caused by pressure on the nerves. Take Venosan and Urticalcin and also make sure that you have sufficient physical exercise. This need not necessarily be strenuous exercise, but every day take a walk in the fresh air.

For several months now I have been suffering from giddiness due to some circulatory problem. It holds me back from leading a full life and going out and about, because I am afraid that it will hit me when least expected.

You will find that taking 15 drops of *Ginkgo biloba* twice daily plus some extra vitamin E will help to stave off these attacks.

My circulation is so bad that I sometimes need resuscitation. What do you think is the best resuscitation method?
The best method of resuscitation is the one outlined in the authorised manual of the British Red Cross:

The ABC of resuscitation

- A is for AIRWAY
  Tilting the casualty's head back and lifting the chin will 'open the airway' – the tilted position lifts the casualty's tongue from the back of the throat so that it does not block the air passage.

- B is for BREATHING
  If a casualty is not breathing, you can breathe for him or her, and thus oxygenate the blood, by giving 'artificial ventilation' blowing your own expelled air into the casualty's lungs.

- C is for CIRCULATION
  If the heart has stopped, 'chest compressions' can be applied to force blood through the heart and around the body. They must be combined with artificial ventilation so that the blood is oxygenated.

COLDS AND CONGESTION

How should one treat a cold – ignore it or do something about it?
Never ignore any distress signals from the body. A cold is a warning that the immune system is being attacked. Always try and bring a cold out, even though it may cause a rise in temperature, or other unpleasant symptoms. Take Echinaforce and plenty of vitamin C because there is nothing to be gained from ignoring a cold.

How would you treat congestion?
Although rarely recognised as such, congestion is a major cause for concern. Statistically, congestion takes more lives than any other disease and it is the body's way of issuing a warning. For congestion of the chest

any one or several of the following remedies are helpful: *Plantago, Petasites, Santasapina*, calcium and vitamin C. For more detailed information read my book *Body Energy*.

CONSTIPATION

What about constipation – is it serious or is it just an inconvenience?
Constipation falls into both categories: it is both serious and a major inconvenience. The bowels play a very important role in the overall body chemistry. Remember the simple rule that whatever is imported, should again be exported within 24 hours. Take good care of your diet and when you do experience such problems use a natural and gentle way to overcome them e.g. use linseed in the form of Linoforce.

My friend is a great believer in regular bowel–cleansing. Is this as good as she makes it out to be?
Many people are not aware that they have a bowel problem and it is especially those people who usually are in greatest need. Often, the whole length of the colon is completely packed with old, hardened faecal matter, leaving only a thin narrow channel which enables small, soft faeces to pass through – commonly called 'tunnel elimination'. Failure to cleanse the colon is like having the entire refuse-collecting staff go on strike for days on end. The colon is the sewage system of the body, but when allowed to stagnate, waste matter will decay and putrify in the blood system, poisoning the brain and nervous system so that you become irritable or depressed, poisoning the heart so that you become weak and listless, poisoning the lungs so that your breath is foul, poisoning the digestive system so that you feel bloated and poisoning the blood so that your skin becomes sallow and unhealthy.

If your diet consists of processed, fried and over-cooked foods, white flour, refined sugar and excessive salt, the colon cannot possibly be efficient, even if you have a bowel movement two or three times a day. Instead of supplying nourishment to the nerves, muscle cells and tissues of the walls of the colon, such foods can actually cause starvation of the colon. A starved colon may let a large amount of faecal matter pass through it, but it is unable to carry out the last stages of digestion. Everyone would benefit by following the recommendations below:

1. Where possible, cut down on processed foods, such as white sugar and white flour.
2. Eat foods that have the least amount of chemical additives, such as artificial food colourings and preservatives.
3. When possible, eat mainly foods that would eventually spoil because they do not contain added preservatives, foods such as fresh fruits and vegetables. Eat a wide variety of vegetables, either raw or cooked in a way that retains most of the nutrients.
4. If you eat frozen foods, use the fluid released in thawing as it often has nutritional value.
5. Avoid a heavy, steady intake of 'junk' food, such as sweets and soft drinks. Where possible, substitute natural sweets and fruit juices.
6. Exercise regularly, taking into consideration your age and general health.

In bowel-cleansing programmes I have read of fasting periods sometimes as long as seven days. Isn't this too long to go without food?

Not really, because in these programmes one should always make sure to drink plenty. This is a time for revitalisation and an effective way to cleanse the body of accumulated wastes and at the same time to rejuvenate the functions of all the vital organs. The body can go without food for long periods of time, but water is essential at all times.

Is it possible that a bowel-cleansing programme or a fasting programme can cause a person to become ill?

Cleansing or fasting can be upsetting if you do not know what to expect. Food withdrawal, especially from coffee, sugar, chocolate or meat can cause headaches and nausea. If you experience these problems, then an enema is especially important to speed the toxins through the system as quickly as possible.

How do you feel about enemas as part of a bowel-cleansing programme?

You should first of all realise that the body, and in this case especially the bowel, needs help. Sometimes an enema is helpful, but the body will still have to do the job itself.

Are colonics helpful as part of a way to overcome constipation?

A good colonic programme can indeed be of great help, but only ever consider using this therapy under expert guidance. It should take no less than thirty minutes and should also include colon massage. Let me, however, point out that this treatment should not be undergone too often.

If drinking water is mentioned in a bowel-cleansing programme, is one allowed to substitute vegetable juices?

By all means, because vegetable juices do not disrupt the healing and rejuvenating process, as is suggested by some water-fast enthusiasts.

Can someone with a wheat allergy take natural wheat bran to combat constipation?

Wheat bran, although a good natural aid for constipation, is not advisable for someone with a diagnosed wheat allergy. Constipation can easily be helped by taking Linoforce granules.

D

DIABETES

Is there an alternative therapy to help diabetes patients?
Yes, alternative medicine can be useful for diabetics, but this should not be considered to the exclusion of professional medical help. Any diabetic condition should be treated with great care. The suitability of any alternative therapy depends on the condition of the individual diabetic patient, and the medication that person requires. However, I have been able to help many diabetics with such therapies, and in quite a few cases we have managed to reduce their insulin dependency. A number of my patients have been able to reverse their condition sufficiently so that it can be kept under control with tablets, whereas they had previously had to inject insulin. In some patients the improvement was such that the condition could be controlled with diet alone.

Diet is always important, but never more so than for diabetics. Cut out sugar altogether and drastically cut down on the intake of carbohydrate. Take Molkosan, which is a milk whey product that encourages the production of more natural insulin. There is also a very good remedy called Myrtillis Complex, containing myrtle and periwinkle. Alternatively, *Nat. sulph. 6x* is excellent, as is an extract of the thin membrane that lines the shells of walnuts. Every day, drink one small glass of this extract, made up as follows: remove the soft kernels from one pound of walnuts and use these in salads. Boil the shells for twenty minutes in sufficient water to cover them and keep this extract in the fridge.

I have continual pain in my legs, which I have been told is because of my diabetic condition. What can you suggest?
Take one 500 IU capsule of vitamin E twice daily and also use a remedy called HypoAde from Enzymatic Therapy. I am sure that soon you will feel better.

What treatment should a diabetic follow? I have been an insulin-user for three or four years now.
Remember that it is never too late. Start as soon as possible by ensuring a healthy and balanced diet. Take Molkosan, Diabetisan and walnut water (see above). Also, eat plenty of leeks and garlic.

Is it true that milk whey can be useful in the treatment of diabetics and, if so, how should it be taken?
Molkosan is a Bioforce product and is produced from fresh Alp whey by a natural fermentation process. It contains all the important minerals found in fresh whey, such as magnesium, potassium and calcium, in concentrated forms. Molkosan is rich in natural dextrorotatory L(+) lactic acid which, in health-oriented nutrition as well as natural healing methods has a special significance. Mix one teaspoon of Molkosan in a glass of water and drink this with every meal of the day.

Could you advise on how to lower the level of blood sugar in diabetes?
Take two capsules of chromium and also 15 drops of Diabetisan, both twice daily. Three times a day take half a teaspoon of Molkosan in half a cup of water, three times a day.

Is it possible to treat hypoglycaemia successfully?
Most definitely! Hypoglycaemia is the opposite condition of diabetes and this can be treated very effectively by eating a high-protein diet. Also use Oil of Evening Primrose.

Can wild leek, Molkosan, Devil's Claw, and raw potato juice as mentioned in your book *Traditional Home and Herbal Remedies*, help an insulin-dependent diabetic?
They most certainly are helpful for the condition you mentioned. I would suggest that diabetics also take Diabetisan and a chromium supplement.

I have neuropathy which, apparently, is caused by diabetes. What should I do?
Take 15 drops of Venosan and one 500 IU capsule of vitamin E twice daily.

I have a spinal stenosis and am also diabetic. The stenosis affects my left leg and my specialist, a neurosurgeon, has said

that I should have an operation. However, I happen to know that it is not a very pleasant operation and I would prefer not to have it and instead treat the pain by natural means or homoeopathic remedies. I have already tried acupuncture for four months and wonder if you have any further suggestions?

I would much prefer to see you for myself, but in general my advice would be to take ten drops of Petaforce and 400 IU of vitamin E twice daily.

Can homoeopathy help for Type I (juvenile) diabetes?

Yes it can, but only ever contemplate using this method under the guidance of a qualified practitioner.

Can you advise me on the treatment for a hyperactive thyroid (for a diabetic) on thyroid-suppressing pills?

Take 15 drops of Nasturtium twice daily.

I have an elderly friend who is 75 years old. Her doctor has diagnosed her as having sugar diabetes, but was unable to give her a diet sheet. How can I obtain one for her?

Any dietician at your local hospital will be able to oblige.

DIARRHOEA

I have diarrhoea almost constantly. What should I do?

This is yet another of those alarm signals mentioned previously which the body emits when there is a physical irregularity. Be very careful because constant diarrhoea may cause dehydration. Study your diet and see if there is something lacking, or alternatively any excess. Read my book *Stomach and Bowel Disorders* for indications. Make sure that your diet contains the correct nutrients to encourage the existence of friendly bacteria in the bowels. If in doubt, eat a helping of natural yoghurt every day or take either *Acidophilus* or *Biodophilus*.

Furthermore, take twice daily 15 drops of Echinaforce before meals and 15 drops of Tormentavena in a little water after meals.

I have suffered for some years now from frequently recurring bouts of diarrhoea. I have had X-rays and have followed various treatment programmes, but without success.

As nothing has come to light as the result of the X-rays, I would suggest that you try some of the advice mentioned above. Your problem is likely to be diet-related.

How can one cope with irritation adjacent to the back passage, coupled with a bad odour?
Drink camomile tea and take 15 drops of Tormentavena in half a cup of water twice daily.

DEPRESSION

What would your advice be for depression?
Depression comes in various forms, e.g. depression as we commonly refer to it, anxiety, stress. You may find that my book *Stress and Nervous Disorders* provides some helpful advice. It is important to find out the cause of the depression and exactly how it affects you. Once these have been determined it will be easier to decide on the method of treatment. It would make sense to consult a doctor, psychiatrist or qualified practitioner.

Are there any homoeopathic preparations that can be used to relieve depression?
Once the correct diagnosis has been made as to the cause of the depression, a qualified practitioner can advise you more specifically. However, the most commonly used remedies are *Sepia 6x, Acid phos. 3x, Ignatia 4x* and *6x, Kalium phos. 6x, Ovarium 3x* and *Nat. mur. 6x*.

I suffer from manic depressive psychosis cycles of extreme lows and highs. I have to take drugs to keep this illness under some control (Maoi-Nardil) plus Largactil when I really cannot sleep when I am on a high. I am allergic to coffee and have an extreme reaction to anything with a high caffeine content. The illness comes in cycles. I don't know what sparks it off (then suddenly it breaks). How can I try and find out how to control it?
When on drugs long-term, such as Nardil, one has to be careful with regard to taking any alternative. You should discuss this further with your doctor and practitioner. My interpretation is that your condition clearly

points to a hormonal imbalance. The highs and lows can be triggered by a number of reasons: an imbalanced diet, the monthly cycle, emotions or shock. You would be well advised to seek the advice of a qualified practitioner.

What is the best herb to use for manic depression?

Sometimes a combination of zinc and valerian helps. Nature's Best also has a remedy that may be useful: Jayvee.

I suffer from depression and severe travel sickness. Can you tell me if there is an alternative remedy for travel sickness?

As a homoeopathic remedy you can use either *Nux vomica* or *Cocculus* for the travel sickness. The depression may be helped by taking Hyperiforce or *Zincum valerianicum*.

Life is so hard for me. Every night when I go to bed I am in a bad mood. When I see that I have done nothing I am so discouraged and depressed that I stay up watching television, because I can change nothing. The time goes so fast and I do nothing. What can I do?

Believe me when I say that watching television until all hours will only make your condition worse. The television screen affects the endocrine system and, as such, lowers the effectiveness of the immune system. Take exercise in the fresh air, such as walking, or cycling, and go swimming Adopting a positive outlook will greatly improve your condition. Read my book *Stress and Nervous Disorders* for more detailed suggestions. Try and force yourself to study the positive things in life and you will find that it is true that behind every cloud a ray of sunshine can be found.

What would you advise for a person who has had depression for years and is not responding to drugs? This person (aged 43) has had to give up work as a result of depression.

My advice would be similar to that given in answer to the previous question. Please read my book *Stress and Nervous Disorders*, because it contains much helpful advice.

What can be done for a chemical imbalance that causes sleeplessness, mixed up dreams and depression?

Of equal importance are checking the diet for imbalances or excesses and learning to relax. Advice on both these measures can be found in my book *Stress and Nervous Disorders*. Remedies such as Neuroforce, Ginsavita, or Jayvee may be of considerable help.

What natural remedies can you recommend for manic depression? Do you think that it can be caused by hormone imbalance? Does having a baby correct this imbalance?

If the cause is indeed due to a hormonal imbalance you will notice a marked improvement during pregnancy. However, this is not a cure, because after the pregnancy the condition may recur. If it is a long-term problem you would be well advised to seek professional medical help from a qualified practitioner. There are many alternative ways in which the condition can be overcome, such as acupuncture, osteopathy, homoeopathy or herbal remedies. As I cannot provide specific advice for your condition without knowing more about your personal circumstances, my advice must be that you seek medical help.

My husband is suffering from nervous anxiety depression. The doctor has advised Diazepam – three times a day. However, I feel that this is making his condition worse. Are there any alternatives he could take?

Many patients who do not react favourably to drugs, respond positively to complementary treatment forms such as acupuncture, osteopathy or herbal remedies. Also, the remedy Kava-Cara has proved to be a good alternative to Diazepam.

Although I know I still care about my family and their problems, I don't seem to feel anything. It is as though only part of me is functioning. The person the outside world sees can hold a conversation and carry on as normal (I work in a bar). At home, most of my time is spent watching television or in bed, as anything else is too much effort. There have been odd times when I have taken a bit of an interest and done some work at home, but only on a few occasions. I will not go out with my husband, who has often suggested that we go swimming or to a movie, which we used to do quite often. I feel so down and depressed, so helpless. I know that I am wasting part of my life, and this condition has lasted for well over two years now. I want to get well and feel alive again,

but feel as though something in my head is stopping me (like a dark cloud blotting out the sun).
It is high time that you did something about this and started to enjoy life again. Life is too good and too sweet to lose a moment of it. Find a good psychologist or natural practitioner and he or she will probably be able to help you to overcome this situation. Positive thinking can work wonders.

Could I have some advice on depression in teenagers? What would you recommend?
It is even harder to understand depression in teenagers, because they have so much to look forward to – if only they knew it. The remedy Hyperiforce will help and, in gerneral, teenagers like my book *Body Energy*, which contains much useful advice.

E

EAR PROBLEMS

My seven-year-old son has an ear infection. What can I do?
Give him five drops of *Plantago* twice daily and also sprinkle five drops of *Plantago* onto a piece of cottonwool and place this deep into the ear during the night. Remove the cottonwool during the day. Usually, the pain will have disappeared within a matter of days.

What can you tell me about the cause and possible treatment for noises in the ear?
Noises in the ears can be caused by many reasons: deafness, tinnitus, Ménière's disease, or other causes. Usually, acupuncture will help and remedies such as *Ginkgo biloba, Plantago* and vitamin B$_3$.

I often have deafness and crackling in the ear, which I feel is caused by catarrh. I have tried *Kali. mur.*, but this has not helped.
I would suggest that you use 20 drops of Echinaforce three times a day.

What would you do about noises in the head? Can this be caused by an allergy or by catarrh?
Specific allergies can indeed affect the ears, but catarrh, a fungus or infections are the more common causes. Consult a qualified practitioner for an accurate diagnosis.

I often have a ringing sensation in the left ear when I turn around quickly. Then my balance becomes affected and I am in danger of falling. What is your advice?
You should have this properly investigated. Possible reasons may be tinnitus, vertigo or Ménière's disease. These complaints can be dealt with

once the correct diagnosis has been made and therefore I would suggest that you consult your doctor or a qualified natural practitioner.

My wife is extremely anxious about her deteriorating hearing. What should she do?

This is one of those instances where acupuncture can often be of great help. Tell your wife that she should take immediate action and seek the help of a qualified acupuncturist.

For five years I have had vertigo, but since I visited your clinic in June 1992 I have not had another attack. Do you think that it will ever return, or am I completely cured?

Very likely it will never recur, but if it does, you must come back immediately.

I am 59 years old and suffer from severe tinnitus in both ears. It is affecting me badly and I wonder if you can advise on how to make this more bearable?

In such cases the correct diagnosis is all-important and after this has been confirmed there are plenty of remedies or therapies that can be used to help. Seek the advice of a qualified practitioner.

Very often, without warning, I feel that my balance is affected. What could be the cause and what, if anything, can be done about it?

This could be caused by vertigo or tinnitus, and in order to prescribe a suitable treatment it is first essential to obtain the correct diagnosis. You need not fear, however, because a qualified practitioner will be able to help you.

What is the treatment for tinnitus?

Tinnitus can be treated with acupuncture, osteopathy, or herbal or homoeopathic treatment. The correct treatment will be decided upon by the practitioner, having taken into account the habits and condition of the individual person concerned.

I am desperate to find a homoeopathic remedy for tinnitus, which affects me badly in my right ear.

Sometimes salicylic acid 6x or *Carb. sulph. D4* is of help. For long-term cases I have often found that *Kalium iod.* 6x has been very effective and if the person is only affected during or after singing, then *China sulph.* 6x is recommended.

Is there any herbal remedy you could advise for my husband, who suffers on and off from tinnitus (ringing in the ears)?
Try him on 15 drops of *Loranthus* twice daily. If this is not successful ask him to make an appointment with a qualified herbal practitioner who should be able to advise him on a more individual treatment method.

Please tell me if tinnitus can be treated and/or cured?
It is always difficult to state categorically that anything can be cured. However, in most cases of tinnitus where I have been consulted, I have been successful in finding a cure, but in a few cases I have failed. You must keep trying and never accept the prognosis that 'You will have to learn to live with it!'

My mother has been told that she suffers from an inner-ear virus called tinnitus, which is said to be incurable. It comes on every two or three days. She has now been advised to use the homoeopathic remedy called *China sulph.* 6x. Can you tell me any more about this?
Your mother has been well advised and if she follows this advice she has already taken a step in the right direction. Personally, I would also advise that twice a day she uses 15 drops of *Loranthus*.

I would like to hear what you would recommend for tinnitus (a recurrent whistling or ringing sound in the ears). I have had a scan, but nothing showed up.
As the scan has shown no reasons for this condition, it might be due to nerve damage. In this case I would advise the use of Oil of Evening Primrose, *Loranthus* and *Ginkgo biloba*.

Please could you give me some recommendations regarding tinnitus. I have constant noises in my head and am also suffering from insomnia.
Indeed, this is a most unpleasant combination: tinnitus as well as insomnia. For both conditions I would suggest that you try the remedies

Avena sativa, *Loranthus* and Dormeasan. If the conditions persist you are well advised to seek the advice of a qualified practitioner.

I suffer from various complaints which to my mind are all related: tinnitus (constant whooshing in the ear), deafness, problems with my balance (dizziness). Some six years ago I was diagnosed as having Ménière's disease. Can you help in any way?

In quite a number of cases like yours I have found that acupuncture has been successful. I would also recommend the use of any of the remedies mentioned in earlier questions on this subject.

ECZEMA

What causes eczema?

Eczema can be caused by a variety of reasons, but few people are aware of the fact that sometimes an allergy to certain plants can be the cause, e.g. primulas or chrysanthemums. Often, asthma is an underlying factor or it is an inherited condition. You may now realise that there can be many reasons for this condition and a qualified practitioner should be able to advise you as to the correct treatment for you as an individual.

My daughter has a rash on her chest which becomes very red and itchy – eczema spots. It seems to be mainly caused by the air. For some time now she has been taking some homoeopathic remedies, but we would be very interested to hear your suggestions about any other forms of medication.

As your daughter has already tried homoeopathic treatment (although you are not specific as to which remedies she has used) I would suggest first of all that she takes Echinaforce and Violaforce (*Viola tricolor*). However, I also feel that she may benefit from a course of vitamins, especially vitamin A.

Our intake of vitamins relies on us being able to extract these vital nutrients from our diet. There are a few exceptions to this, for example vitamin D can be synthesised within the skin, but overall, the definition of a vitamin is that adequate amounts can only be supplied in the diet.

Vitamins are essential for health and if any one of the thirteen recognised vitamins was to be missing from our diet, it would be unlikely to leave us unaffected. The function of vitamins is closely linked with that of enzymes, which are essential chemicals, produced by the body. There are thousands of different enzymes in the body, most of which are within the cells and tissues, where they control biochemical reactions. Both the rate and results of these reactions rely on the presence of these enzymes, which themselves rely on substances called co-enzymes, to literally 'switch them on and off'. Co-enzymes are vitamins or derivatives produced from a vitamin. It is through this control mechanism that vitamins exert such great effect and play such a vital role, despite the minute quantities in which they are required.

There are two main groups of vitamins – water-soluble and fat-soluble. Water-soluble vitamins consist of the B vitamins and vitamin C. They tend to have a short life in the body, with little storage taking place. On the other hand, the fat-soluble vitamins A, D, E and K are stored in the body.

Vitamins are easily lost from our food by the processes of peeling, freezing and cooking and it is possible to lose up to 90 per cent of available vitamins in this way if food is poorly stored and overcooked. Vitamin A occurs in nature in two forms, as retinol and as carotene. Retinol is the only preformed vitamin A available from dietary sources and can only be found in foods of animal, fish or poultry origin, such as liver and fish oils. It is produced by these animals from carotene. Carotene is found in green vegetables and carrots, and our bodies are also able to convert it into vitamin A.

Vitamin A plays an important role in the health of many tissues and helps to maintain a smooth, soft, healthy skin. Internally, it helps to maintain the mucous membranes of the lungs, throat, nose and mouth. These tissues protect our bodies from the environment and are responsible for trapping any particles and micro-organisms that are inhaled. Tiny microscopic hairs, or cilia, present on the surface of the membranes move the particles out of the lungs to where they can be safely swallowed.

Vitamin A is used by the thymus gland – the key organ of the immune system – and it is also involved in the formation of our blood, bones and teeth. It is essential for keeping the eyes healthy and moist and forms part of the light-sensitive pigments of the eyes, where it is required for optimum night vision. Over 90 per cent of the body's vitamin A is stored in the liver, and an adequate supply of zinc is needed to enable the liver to mobilise these reserves.

What diet would you recommend for the treatment of eczema?

In all cases of eczema I would advise the reduction or elimination of citrus fruits, dairy foods and pork in any shape or form. For more detailed dietary advice please read my book *Skin Diseases*.

How should chronic eczema be treated?
It should be realised that eczema can have a number of underlying causes. Once the cause has been determined it will be possible to decide upon the appropriate treatment. It is often overlooked too, that there are several kinds of eczema, to name but a few: contact eczema, detergent eczema, infantile eczema and discoid eczema. In order to advise on the treatment therefore, a correct diagnosis should be obtained.

Can you please advise on an external treatment for eczema. My daughter is greatly bothered with spots which are said to originate from an eczema condition.
For external treatment I can suggest any one of the following creams: Bioforce's 7 Herb Cream, Violaforce cream or vitamin E cream.

What is the cause of infantile eczema?
This condition occurs when previously breast-fed babies have been weaned and are given cows' milk instead. It should be remembered that cows' milk contains nine times more protein than mothers' milk and often the baby is unable to cope with the increased protein intake. In such cases asthma or eczema may occur. The use of Violaforce (extract of the wild pansy) is helpful, together with Oil of Evening Primrose and Bioforce's 7 Herb Cream.

My 12-month-old granddaughter suffers from infantile eczema. She is very distressed and constantly scratching, to the point of drawing blood. Her entire body is covered with the rash and the prescribed medication has brought about no improvement. Have you any suggestions?
The child's mother should be advised to read my book *Skin Diseases* for dietary information. She can also safely give the child five drops of *Viola tricolor* twice daily.

My seven-month-old daughter has extremely dry skin and has patches of eczema or psoriasis, especially on her face and hands. She is on soya formula and eats only the foods a seven-

months-old should eat. One paediatrician told me to be aggressive with 1 per cent cortisone and Benedryl. I hate to do it. Do you think it is genetic or can diet change the dryness of the skin?

I sympathise with you and concur that steroid cortisone is the last thing one should use. There are so many alternatives that should first be tried. Especially with what are, after all, minor problems (although I agree that they are irksome, and should be cleared) such aggressive methods should be avoided. Please read my book *Skin Diseases* for more detailed advice.

How would you advise an eczema sufferer who would like to do more than just keep this bothersome condition under control with creams and ointments? I take Oil of Evening Primrose capsules and am careful to avoid artificial flavourings and colourings in my diet.

You already have taken some very sensible steps, but you may well require some more remedial assistance. Try some of the homoeopathic or herbal remedies and therapies mentioned in my book *Skin Diseases*.

What diet should one follow for helping eczema and psoriasis? Also, please tell me what herbal creams are available for this purpose.

For general dietary instructions please read my book *Skin Diseases*. As for the second part of your question, it should be realised that the skin is a vital, highly complex system which performs many functions. Not least, it acts as a barrier to protect the internal organs from damage and infection, regulates the body temperature, eliminates waste fluid and acts as a trigger to our senses between our bodies and the environment. Alcohol, smoking, lack of sleep, busy life styles, poor diet, environmental pollution and the elements – cold, wind and the sun – ali affect the appearance and health of our skin. With this in mind, Nature's Best have introduced a unique range of special skin-care products specifically designed to combat the ravages of the environment. From this range I have selected two which may be of help to you.

Aloe Vera/Vitamin E Cream: This moisturising cream helps to protect the skin from the rigours of city life and the punishment it receives from the sun, wind and cold. It softens and replenishes the skin and at the same time provides a considerable source of vitamin E. Rich in soothing and refreshing aloe vera gel, this cream may help to protect and improve the appearance of the skin. The cream is hypo-allergenic and suitable for all the family.

NaPCA Moisturiser: This cream, which contains eucalyptus, is a pH-balanced concentrated solution of the sodium salt of pyrrolidone carboxylix acid (NaPCA), the most important natural moisturising factor found in human skin. The substance NaPCA draws water out of the air, moisturising the skin and improving its appearance. Although it is produced by the body, we lose up to 50 per cent as we age, reducing our ability to keep our skin soft and moist.

Nature's Best's NaPCA Cream is safe to use on either the face or the body and will help to protect the skin from drying out in the sun, wind or equally hostile indoor environments such as central heating. It is also popular with men, who find it helps to prevent flaking of the skin after shaving.

What is the best remedy for eczema? My son is 18 years of age now and he has had it since he was 18 months old.
Unless I was able to see your son I could only advise in general. Read my book on *Skin Diseases* for dietary advice and suggested herbal remedies.

My daughter suffers badly from very dry skin on her hands, and eczema. She has tried Betnovate and E45 cream, but neither of these has been successful. Do you have any suggestions?
The treatment for eczema and dry skin should be both internal and external. Dry skin eczema usually reacts well to the herbal remedies *Viola tricolor* or Violaforce and Oil of Evening Primrose. For homoeopathic remedies I would suggest *Aluminia 6x* or *Arsenicum 6x*. For external use try either one of these two ointments: Bioforce 7 Herb Cream or Echinacea Cream. Tell your daughter not to give up.

Can you advise me on herbal and/or homoeopathic treatments for eczema please?
Suitable homoeopathic remedies for eczema are *Graphites D6, Sulphur 6x, Rhus tox, Hepar sulph.* and *Psorinum.*

Among herbal remedies I would include *Viola tricolor* and Echinaforce. For dry eczema try blue flag root, while for moist eczema I would suggest red clover.

Would you please advise on general treatment methods and remedies for eczema and tell me if it is possible that stress can influence the condition?

You are quite right, stress is an influential factor in eczema and psoriasis. Read my book *Skin Diseases* for advice on general treatment methods and I would suggest that you also read my book *Stress and Nervous Disorders*, paying special attention to the section on Hara breathing exercises.

Can you recommend anything at all for dry eczema on the face and scalp? As yet I have not found anything that is fully effective.

Many of my patients have been very pleased with the results when using Skin and Hair and Skin Nutrition capsules from Vita Biotics.

Is there anything which can be done to ease eczema on the feet and hands only? It has been diagnosed as being caused by nerves. My 32-year-old son suffers badly with this and the condition only developed some three years ago. I would so much like to help him.

If the condition has limited itself so far to the hands and feet I would suggest the remedy Petaforce. Three times a week, before going to bed, rub the affected areas with castor oil and loosely dress the oiled extremities with soft cotton gloves or socks, covered if necessary with plastic or cellophane to allow this oil to penetrate overnight without soiling the bed clothes.

Can skin conditions such as acne and eczema be treated with homoeopathic medicines?

A wholehearted 'Yes' is my answer to your question and I would suggest that you read my book *Skin Diseases* for more detailed information.

I follow a good wholefood diet and drink spring water, and yet I still suffer from eczema. What do you suggest?

I am pleased to hear that you are taking a sensible approach, because diet is a very important factor. However, you should also try some homoeopathic or herbal remedies and I am sure that you will find some suitable advice for your specific condition in my book *Skin Diseases*.

Can you suggest some treatment – homoeopathic or herbal – for a cat with chronic eczema (the vet says that it is caused by a hormone imbalance)?

Domestic pets, such as cats and dogs, can also be treated by herbal, homoeopathic or vitamin therapies, and Oil of Evening Primrose capsules are often of great help. As for your specific request I can tell you about two remedies that have been specifically designed for this purpose, i.e. HiVitimin for Cats and HiVitimin for Dogs. Both have been formulated by a veterinary surgeon, and are concentrated vitamin and mineral supplements presented as granules for mixing with the pet's food. Most breeders accept this as being the best way to improve an animal's diet and they have little time for the low-potency supplements in the form of tablets, which are often little more than 'treats'. By adding supplements to your pet's food you can be sure they will eat it. More details on these remedies are given below:

HiVitimin for Dogs: This is a highly palatable powder which is mixed with the dog's food. It contains 28 essential nutrients at sensible levels and is believed to be by far the most comprehensive supplement for dogs available. All dogs can be given HiVitimin, including show dogs and pregnant and lactating bitches.

HiVitimin for Cats: This is a superb product, containing 29 active ingredients presented in a palatable form that cats take to easily. Although tinned cat food is usually high enough in protein to satisfy all protein needs, it is nevertheless not the same as the fresh (uncooked) meat or fish which cats would eat in the wild. The high-temperature processing that tinned food undergoes can destroy some of the vitamin content of the food. A regular addition of HiVitimin to the cat's diet will ensure that the animal receives a high level of vitamins and minerals. HiVitimin for cats also contains the amino acid Taurine because it is essential that it is present in the pet's diet. Humans and other animals such as dogs do not need this amino acid as it can be made within the body.

EMPHYSEMA

Is it possible to treat emphysema or must one accept that it is a 'hopeless' condition?

Nothing should ever be seen as 'hopeless'. Nature wants to cure! However, emphysema is not an easy condition to relieve because the air sacs become enlarged and rupture. If breathing requires effort or is forced, these air sacs will stretch and may eventually burst. It is true that this condition cannot be 'cured', although it is certainly possible to maintain a measure of control by herbal treatment and natural antibiotics.

The first rule is *no smoking*, of course, and plenty of fresh air. In addition, use vitamin E, Irish moss, Echinaforce and ASM Drops. Dairy foods, where possible, should be avoided.

Briefly, how would you treat emphysema?
Depending upon the condition of the patient, variably by acupuncture, osteopathy, herbal treatment and diet. I would also strongly recommend the Hara breathing exercises, as described in my book *Stress and Nervous Disorders*.

What advice on herbal or homoeopathic treatment would you give to an emphysema patient?
Twice daily, take 15 drops of ASM Drops before meals and one 500 IU capsule of vitamin E after meals.

ENTERITIS

What can be done about enteritis?
The golden rule is to follow a balanced diet, and guidelines for this can be found in my book *Stomach and Bowel Disorders*. Also, the remedy *Centaurium* should be taken twice daily (15 drops, before meals).

EPILEPSY

Is it true that epilepsy is a form of headache or migraine?
Indeed, a very bad migraine can be almost a form of epilepsy. Sometimes in such cases the diagnosis is borderline: a migraine or an epileptic attack. At such times *Loranthus* is the best recommendation.

I have been told that a naturopath will investigate the cause, rather than treat the symptoms. What causes epilepsy?

Epilepsy can be brought about through trauma and/or miasmas. It can also be due to a hereditary factor or stress conditions. My book *Migraine and Epilepsy* may give you a better understanding of this condition.

Can epilepsy be cured or overcome?
The ability to cure a condition such as epilepsy is a claim that is difficult to substantiate. However, I have often seen impressive results obtained with homoeopathic, herbal or vitamin therapies.

My husband was diagnosed as suffering from epilepsy when he was 22 years old. He takes several drugs, but we often wonder if there are any homoeopathic remedies available for this condition?
In many cases I have seen patients use homoeopathic remedies alongside the drugs prescribed by their specialist, and eventually the drug intake could be reduced while the condition remained stable.

My 13-year-old son has epilepsy. Can it be treated by homoeopathy – or by anti-convulsants combined with homoeopathy? If so, does it require co-operation from the patient, as my son is reluctant to help himself, e.g. I have to insist on no cheese and chocolate as they do not seem to agree with him.
Your son must learn to accept the importance of dietary management for his condition. My book *Migraine and Epilepsy* explains how homoeopathic and herbal remedies can sometimes help to reduce the intake of drugs.

My grandson, aged 24, has epilepsy and recently has had several fits. He has been taking various medications, which have not really seemed to help. He has now been referred to a neurologist, but is worried about what this involves. Can you help in any way?
I can understand that you are somewhat concerned, but remember that it is always best to have any condition properly investigated. If a specific diagnosis is reached, your grandson might benefit greatly. I must repeat that alternative treatment is often very helpful, especially if it means that the drug intake can be reduced. It is even possible in some cases to eliminate all drugs and to replace them with homoeopathic or herbal remedies. However, this should only ever be considered in conjunction with your grandson's doctor, and never without proper medical guidance.

Can stress cause epileptic attacks?
If one is susceptible to this condition, it is quite possible that attacks can be brought on by stress.

What treatment would you recommend for complex partial seizures, equilibrium problems and vertigo?
I would strongly suggest two homoeopathic remedies: *Cerebrum* and *Loranthus.* However, I must stress that if you experience these problems, I sincerely hope that you are under regular medical supervision.

EXHAUSTION

What would you suggest for exhaustion?
Depending on the condition of the person concerned and upon the circumstances, there are a variety of remedies to choose from, such as *Ginkgo biloba*, Ginsavita, Imuno-Strength and Neuroforce. You should also read the questions and answers under the heading 'Nervous complaints and disorders'.

EYE PROBLEMS

My eyes are often inflamed. What can I do?
Inflammation of the eyes is often due to other problems. You should consult your doctor or practitioner. Sometimes an eye wash prepared using half a teaspoon of Epsom salts or with Euphrasia officinalis (eyebright) is beneficial, as are camomile compresses.

What would you recommend for floaters in the eyes, i.e. a small speck that is hardly noticeable, but always there?
It is possible that your blood circulation is not what it should be. Try taking 15 drops of Arterioforce, together with 4 tablets of Urticalcin, both twice daily.

Please can you suggest a remedy for dry eyes?
Take ten drops of Euphrasia officinalis twice daily.

I always seem to have dry eyes, mouth and nose. I have tried artificial tears, but found these of little help. I would very much like to take a computer course and have been told that

this could aggravate my complaints. Can you help?

Computers, wordprocessors and televisions are never considered advantageous for the eyes, as any VDU (visual display unit) is likely to produce eye strain and dryness. If much time is spent – whether it be in the line of work or your spare time watching a VDU screen, ensure that you also take plenty of outdoor exercise: walking, swimming or cycling. Also to help this condition you should add a few drops of Euphrasia officinalis and some Epsom salts to some warm water and use this for a good eyewash. Take plenty of vitamin A and Urticalcin.

What can one do about occasional blood vessel ruptures on the whites of the eyes (possibly every few months or so)?

Take 15 drops of Hyperisan in half a cup of water twice daily.

Can you offer any advice on treatment for dry mouth and eyes? I have been told this is Sjörgen's disease and that there is very little to be done about it.

Taking one dessertspoon of codliver oil before going to bed is often helpful. I would suggest that you also take three capsules of Oil of Evening Primrose daily.

Please tell me if it is possible to prevent cataracts?

Unless there are other conditions involved, my general advice would be to take one or two tablets of Health Insurance Plus daily. It would also be wise to take some extra calcium and therefore I would suggest taking four tablets of Urticalcin and two *Silicea* tablets twice daily.

My husband got a laser beam or some chemical in his eye. He is unsure what exactly happened, but his eyesight has been affected and he also has some pain in the eye.

If the condition was triggered by a laser beam, the condition will be especially aggravated in the early stages. He would be wise to take supplementary vitamins, minerals and trace elements.

My sister suffers from dry eyes and mouth, and also gets conjunctivitis and swollen eyelids. She uses an eye lubricant and bathes her eyes in saline. Is there anything you can recommend?

Conjunctivitis is caused by inflammation of the conjunctiva, which is mostly caused by an infection or allergy. This condition can be quickly cleared by using an eyewash prepared with diluted Euphrasia officinalis and eyedrops called Oculosan.

My mother would like to know if there is anything you could recommend for lines and circles around the eyes?
Use an oil-based cream externally and, to ensure that the kidneys function optimally, take Oil of Evening Primrose capsules.

I would be grateful for some advice on treatment for burning eyes.
Use camomile compresses, vitamin E or Occulosan eyedrops.

Could the reason for suffering sore and gritty eyes be stress-related or might there be some other underlying cause?
This problem is probably caused by artificial lighting. I am sure that taking ten drops of Euphrasia officinalis twice daily will help greatly.

Since sitting a diploma last year I have continually suffered from itchy, red, swollen eyes, which normally flare up in the morning. The swelling lasts for one or two days and the eyes then remain red and itchy and the surrounding skin becomes flaky for around a week. This normally happens when I am feeling under stress, but not always. I have been to the doctor several times and have had HC45 cream prescribed, but I really do not think it does any good.
This is not an unusual aftermath for a period of stress. Once such a condition has taken hold, it somehow forgets to stop. Twice daily, take 20 drops of Echinaforce before meals and ten drops of Euphrasia officinalis after meals.

Can you recommend any remedies or therapies to improve the eyesight?
Try using Imuno-Strength, Urticalcin and eyebright. However, to find out if there are specific reasons which may be the cause of failing eyesight, please consult your doctor or practitioner.

Would you please tell me how cataracts can be treated?
There are two types of cataracts: grey and green cataracts. For grey

cataracts take ten drops of Arterioforce twice daily. For green cataracts take ten drops of Venosan twice daily. In both cases you should also take four tablets of Urticalcin twice a day.

I have been wearing plastic contact lenses for ten years, but recently I have noticed some discomfort and have therefore gone back to wearing spectacles. What is your view on the long-term effect of wearing contact lenses?
Modern contact lenses are extremely good, but occasionally their long-term use can cause a few problems. If you would like to try your lenses again, also use a good eyewash every morning and evening.

Do you think the wearing of soft contact lenses is safe, or do you have reservations?
Whether one wears contact lenses or spectacles, I agree in either case it is a nuisance. However, no one wears them unless they are needed. If soft contact lenses do not cause any problem to the wearer, they are certainly much more convenient than wearing spectacles and I cannot see any cause for concern.

Having tried four different medications, I have been unable to clear up an eye infection. Is this because my immune system is low, or is there an alternative treatment method?
Your lack of success in overcoming an eye infection could indeed be due to an impaired immune system, but it is also likely that it is as a result of an allergy. Take 20 drops of Echinaforce and two tablets of Imuno-Strength twice daily.

Could you suggest any treatment for my son, who suffers from eye strain caused by working at a light table all day in the printing trade? He has also had conjunctivitis.
I have already mentioned the adverse effects of VDUs on the eyes; the effect of working at a light table is very similar. Advise your son to take supplementary vitamins, minerals and trace elements, because this will strengthen the eyes. Wheatgerm and Imuno-Strength are also recommended.

I have anaemia, which appears to have affected my eyes. I now suffer from severe headaches which seem to originate

from the eyeball sockets and spread to the side of my head and then to the back. Can you confirm that this is indeed related to the coroid anaemia condition? I would also appreciate any advice you can give me.

You are right, because such a connection is not uncommon. Make sure to seek treatment for the anaemia, but also treat the eyes. Take four tablets of Alfavena twice daily and eat plenty of carrots and beetroot.

Is there a herbal remedy that is suitable for the treatment of red veins in the eyes?

Take 15 drops of Venosan in half a cup of water twice daily.

I have been diagnosed as having 'late stage closed-angle ice glaucoma', which apparently is hard to treat. Surgery may help, but what about herbal treatment – is this possible?

Glaucoma is caused by the build-up of fluids in the eye, between the cornea and the lens. Blockage of the channel between the iris and the cornea is known as angle-closure glaucoma. Sometimes 'ice glaucoma' responds well to laser treatment. All glaucoma conditions benefit from supplementary vitamin C and a wholesome diet (liver should be included). Also, use Imuno-Strength to supplement your intake of vitamins.

In late-diagnosed glaucoma, where my physician recommends surgery, is there a herbal remedy that can help to overcome this condition and so avoid an operation?

Unfortunately, glaucoma operations are not as widely successful as cataract operations. Read my response to the previous question and be sure to take additional vitamin C.

F

FATIGUE

I seem to be constantly tired out and always without energy. Can you give me any general advice on how to overcome fatigue?
Some very good advice can be found in my book *Body Energy*. In general, I would suggest a choice of any of the following remedies: Hyssop tincture, Ginsavena or *Ginkgo biloba*.

What do you recommend for a 25-year-old female who complains of being tired and lacking energy?
Take one tablet of Imuno-Strength twice daily.

FOOT PROBLEMS

How can I combat excessive perspiration of the feet?
It is not advisable to entirely eliminate perspiration of the feet, because perspiration is one of the body's methods for the disposal of waste material. However, to take the smell away there is a very old remedy I learned when I was still a student. Buy some borax powder, which is available at most chemists, and once a week or so sprinkle a small quantity in your shoes. You will find that you have to do this less and less frequently, e.g. at intervals of one month or even less. Another benefit is that the skin of the feet will feel much more supple.

For the reduction of perspiration in general, take twice daily 15 drops of Nephrosolid in a cup of Golden Grass Tea. You may also use the well-known cooking herb sage (or *Salvia*). This remedy is available in drops and 15 drops should be taken twice daily before meals.

I am male and 76 years old. I know that my diet leaves something to be desired, but surely this cannot be the cause of my foot problems. I suffer very badly from burning feet and this tires me unduly in the afternoon and evening.

Burning feet generally are an indication of an impaired blood circulation. Supplementary vitamin E is often found to be helpful. You may not know that vitamin E is the most powerful anti-oxidant vitamin in the body. Its prime function is to help scavenge highly reactive free radicals, which are by-products of oxygen metabolism. In nature, vitamin E occurs as tocopherols, of which there are four forms. The most biologically potent form is d-alpha tocopherol, which is 100 per cent biologically active.

In practice, the name vitamin E refers to the d-alpha tocopherol form. It is a yellow oil that is insoluble in water but soluble in fats and oils. Like the other fat-soluble vitamins, A, D and K, vitamin E is transported around the body dissolved in fats and is stored in fatty tissue to be used when it is needed.

Vitamin E occurs naturally in cereals, vegetable oils, raw seeds, nuts and soya beans. It is also added to certain prepared foods, such as polyunsatured margarine, to help prevent the oil going rancid.

Vitamin E protects polyunsatured fats from becoming oxidised, and hence promotes the proper functioning of fatty acids such as linolenic acid. It also protects other vitamins (A, B-complex and C) as well as both the pituitary and adrenal hormones from being oxidised. The protective effect that vitamin E has on polyunsatured fats results in the vitamin being used up. Thus the more polyunsatured fats that are consumed, the more vitamin E is necessary. Vitamin E is known to have an essential role in cellular respiration where it helps to ensure that oxygen is used efficiently by the blood and muscles; for this reason it is favoured by sports people working to increase their stamina. This important vitamin is also involved in the control of the blood-clotting mechanisms of the body, and it plays a part in the maintenance of healthy capillary walls and the integrity of the red blood cells.

Can you possibly help with fungus problems on the feet?

Internally, *Psorinum*, which is a homoeopathic remedy, and Petaforce should be taken. For external treatment I would advise that *Spilanthes* is dabbed onto the affected areas at regular intervals.

FLATULENCE

What can you advise to curb or control flatulence? I am sometimes so embarrassed when I have problems in company, but I do not know how to reduce it.

Flatulence is no more than alarm bells indicating that the digestive process is not quite what it should be. Digestion is one thing, but absorption is another. Don't ignore flatulence, but check that your diet is adequate. Also, some natural remedies may help, e.g. peppermint capsules, Gastronol and Gastrosan.

Flatulence is often an indication of an enzyme shortage. Enzymes are produced within all living cells and function as catalysts in biochemical reactions. Most enzymes remain with the cells, but in the case of digestive enzymes they are secreted into the digestive tract where they break up food into molecules that are small enough to be absorbed from the gut into the blood stream.

Digestive enzymes are divided into several groups, depending on the type of food substances they act on. For example, lipases act on fats, amylases on starch and proteases on protein. Enzymes are very sensitive to their environment, and can be inactivated by extreme acidity or alkalinity. Our natural production of enzymes may decline as we age, and smokers, drinkers and those who consume a lot of processed foods, often choose to take a digestive enzyme supplement.

As we age hydrochloric acid production in the stomach is reduced, but it remains important for the efficient breakdown of food in the gut. Hydrochloric acid has several different functions in this respect: it helps to sterilise the ingested food and to maintain the correct pH balance in the stomach and it also activates pepsin, the protein-splitting enzyme produced in the stomach. The elderly, people with hectic life styles and others who wish to ensure a sufficiency of hydrochloric acid, may choose to take this supplement.

One of the traditional standbys of natural health practitioners, charcoal, is noted for its ability to absorb internal gases, while passing undigested through the system. A more modern method is the remedy Pineapple Chews from Nature's Best. These are pleasant chewable tablets based on the exotic fruits papaya and pineapple, which supply the natural digestive enzymes papain and bromelain. These enzymes digest proteins, starches and other carbohydrates. Sports people on high-protein diets may choose to use this remedy.

G

GALLBLADDER PROBLEMS

Is it possible to get rid of gallstones without surgery?
Indeed, one should always initially avoid an operation for gallstones, because there are many homoeopathic remedies to help the body rid itself of gallstones, e.g. *Berberis Taraxacum off.* and *Boldocynara*. Also many of my patients have found relief with the help of a very old remedy, which involves drinking half a pint of olive oil in one go. I know that this cannot be an easy task, but if the patient manages to drink half a pint of oil, the oil does not enter the gallbladder, but merely stimulates the secretion of bile which will carry the small and medium stones with it. Before starting this oil cure, artichokes and other herbal remedies should be taken in order to liquefy the gall. As the bowels should be thoroughly cleansed, it is recommended that the patient eat some soaked prunes or figs. If this does not induce the required effect, an enema of warm water with camomile should be used. When the bowels are empty the half pint of olive oil can be drunk and hot packs should be placed over the liver area for two hours before and two hours after drinking the oil.

Lie down on the right side for two hours. If it proves impossible to drink the oil by itself or in one go, it may be mixed with coffee or it may be drunk at intervals. This will be somewhat less effective, but will still cleanse the liver and the smaller stones will come away, although the bigger stones will be left behind. These, however, may be less bothersome for a while. If the patient is capable of drinking the oil all at once, the bigger stones may also be flushed away.

If the situation has become chronic, surgery may indeed be the only answer, but the oil cure has proved very satisfactory in many cases and there is no doubt that this is a preferable method to surgery and its after-effects.

I suspect that I have gallstones and wonder if there are any risks involved in taking the oil cure I have read about in your book _Traditional Home and Herbal Remedies?_

There is no risk involved in the oil cure and you may be very pleasantly surprised by the eventual outcome. Please do not be put off by a feeling of sickness you may experience while undergoing the cure, because, as you can imagine, that will pass.

I have gallbladder trouble of fairly long standing. What items of food should be restricted or avoided?

Avoid all fatty foods and follow the liver diet, as outlined on pages 150-1.

Since I had my gallbladder removed some four years ago I still have a pain where my liver is. I cannot tolerate fat and would like your advice on diet.

In your case I would strongly advise that you take, twice daily, two Temoe Lawak tablets, derived from the Indian herb _Rhizoma curcumae javanica._ Alternatively, try two tablets of Daoen Remoekdjoeng, yet another Indian remedy.

The non-function of my gallbladder was diagnosed in 1981, when I decided against an operation for its removal. I have kept to a fat-free diet, which has greatly helped my condition. Recently, however, I do not seem to be able to control my problems by diet alone. For all these years my diet has been mostly vegetarian, apart from chicken and fish. What would you suggest?

This sounds to me like congestion of the gallbladder and I would recommend that you use the naturopathic remedy _Berberis vulgaris_ (15 drops twice daily).

GLANDS

What should I do if my neck glands are swollen?

Always consult your doctor, because the neck glands do not swell up without an underlying reason. Usually if the neck glands are swollen as well as the under-arm and upper-leg glands, the problem involves the lymph glands. A detoxifying programme should then be considered. In such cases Dr Vogel's Detox Box Programme is highly recommended.

I have a sixteen-year-old daughter who has been troubled with swollen and lumpy glands in her neck and under her arms. Swabs have been taken by our GP and no infection is present. Our doctor advises paracetamol, which is of no help at all. Her condition has been troubling her for approximately two years. She has had reflexology treatment, which has been partly successful. We would appreciate any suggestions.

Reflexology was indeed a sensible step to take, but also try some homoeopathic remedies such as *Sulph. tod. 6x, Fucus ves. 3x, Calcara phosph. 6x, Kalium iod. 4x* or *Conium mac. 4x.*

GUM DISEASE

What, if anything, can be done about inflammation of the gums?

Inflamed gums will benefit greatly from *Propolis*. This can be used internally as well as externally. Also for external use a handy *Propolis* gel is available that can be massaged onto the gums.

Would you please advise me what I should do about bleeding gums?

Often this problem points to a deficiency of vitamin C. Start as soon as possible by taking 2 g of vitamin C daily and twice daily rub some *Propolis* gel onto the gums.

H

HAEMORRHOIDS

Is there a cure for haemorrhoids? With the use of cream I can relieve the pain, but the actual condition is not cured, because the symptoms recur.
Haemorrhoids are caused by blood circulatory problems and for general advice I would suggest that you read the relevant section in this book and also my book *Heart and Blood Circulatory Disorders*. I would recommend that you take 20 drops of *Aesculus hipp.* twice daily, before meals, together with five Urticalcin tablets. In persistent cases also take 15 drops of Venosan twice daily after meals.

What should I do about bleeding haemorrhoids?
As with the previous question, general advice can be obtained from my book on circulatory disorders. In cases of bleeding haemorrhoids I would suggest you take ten drops of *Hamamelis virg.* (witch hazel) twice daily.

My mother suffers badly from haemorrhoids and has tried everything. Can you advise her?
I have found that elderly people, especially, obtain relief by taking, twice daily, 15 drops of *Hamamelis virg.* before meals and 15 drops of Venosan after meals.

HAIR AND SCALP PROBLEMS

Can anything be done about hair loss?
In order to answer your question correctly I would need to know where the hair loss occurs. If the hair thinning or loss is on the front it may be due to atmospheric or hormonal influences, depending on the individual

circumstances, while loss of hair on the middle of the head is usually due to hormonal conditions and hair loss at the back of the head is largely due to an inherited factor. When patches of hair loss are spread over the scalp, the cause is usually an infection. Hair loss in general can often be due to a deficiency of calcium, silicium or vitamins. For general cases I would recommend Urticalcin. Liver cleansing with Boldocynara is always beneficial, as are wheatgerm capsules. If you are concerned, please consult a qualified practitioner who may be able to help you with advice that is more specific to your condition.

I have a very itchy scalp – it is very crusty and flakes off. I have started to use Biosthetic shampoo, which is helping slightly, but I would be grateful if you could suggest anything else that might be of help.
The condition you describe is often indicative of a vitamin A deficiency. Eat plenty of raw carrots and take a vitamin A supplement. Wash your hair with Dr Vogel's Stinging Nettle Hair Lotion.

I am 48 years old and some six months ago the front part of my hair fell out. I have been to a specialist and have been told that it is not alopecia. Can you please help?
This is quite possibly due to a hormonal condition. Try Urticalcin and Oil of Evening Primrose capsules. Take five tablets of Urticalcin twice daily and before going to bed take three capsules of Oil of Evening Primrose. The latter remedy is especially good for hormonal imbalances. This plant – *Oenothera biennis* – has large fragrant flowers which bloom in the early evening, hence the name 'evening primrose'. It is often found growing wild, although it is now extensively cultivated for the seeds that yield the oil.

Research has revealed that the oil is exceptionally high in gamma linolenic acid (GLA), a substance with an essential role in the production of certain hormones (prostaglandins) which regulate many body functions such as blood pressure and the reproductive cycle. Many women choose to take a supplement of evening primrose oil around the time of their period or when going through the menopause.

Although the body can produce GLA directly from an essential fatty acid (EFA) called linolenic acid, sometimes the conversion is not very efficient, so a dietary source may be useful. As nutrients, essential fatty acids are as important as vitamins and minerals, but they cannot be made in the body and have to be supplied in our food. Human breast milk is one of the richest sources of GLA but experts have now identified a more convenient source – evening primrose oil.

It is best if the seeds from the evening primrose plant are pressed to extract the oil using a 'cold' process (as opposed to one that involves heat). Apart from taking Oil of Evening Primrose orally as a food supplement, the precious oil contained within each capsule can also be used to enrich and care for dry skin and hair loss.

My hair is falling out, but my doctor says that I do not have alopecia. The recommended B complex vitamins do not seem to have any impact.
Very often stress and emotion over-taxes the liver. Take ten drops of Boldocynara after meals twice daily. Also consider using some extra Urticalcin and the Hair Formula from Nature's Best.

Do you have an effective treatment or remedy for alopecia? If need be I can follow a specialised diet, although if it is too time-consuming it will not fit in with my life style. I don't think that I am particularly nervous.
Complete alopecia is very difficult to treat. However, there are also cases where I have seen complete recovery. Sometimes good results are obtained with Priorin – a Swiss formula. You could also try acupuncture or electro-frequency treatment. It should also be remembered that smoking, drinking and lack of rest or sleep do have an effect on the condition of one's hair and on the regular growth of hair.

Does prematurely grey hair indicate a health problem?
Premature greying could well be due to hereditary causes, but it could also indicate a zinc deficiency. If in doubt, please take 50 mg of zinc twice daily.

Can you recommend anything to avoid the greying of hair?
Some people have been able to keep premature greying within bounds by taking 50 mg of zinc twice daily. If you are perturbed about the greying of your hair, you may consider the use of some natural and herbal dyes that are not detrimental to the condition of the hair.

I have alopecia for the second time in my life and believe it is connected to an emotional shock and then further stress. Is stress linked to hair loss?

It is not unusual for shock or stress to cause hair loss. The liver is greatly subject to stress and at such moments does not provide the hair root with enough nutrition to help its growth and development.

Can you advise on the thinning of hair? Much hair falls out when it is being washed. It is quite thick as far as my shoulder level, from where it grows much thinner.
It is quite normal to loose 40–60 hairs a day, although we are rarely aware of that. If the hair loss is in excess of this you should try and help the condition with supplementary vitamins, minerals and trace elements.

I have a scalp disorder for which there is no cure, so I have been told. Can you offer help?
If this scalp disorder is caused by excessive dandruff displaying itself as a skin disorder, massage the scalp with Dr Vogel's Onion Hair Lotion. However, first make sure that the condition is properly diagnosed.

My son, who is a student, suffers from *Alopecia areata* in his beard and hair. We would be interested to know if a vitamin supplement would help?
Advise your son to take one tablet of Hair Factor from Nature's Best three times daily.

HAY FEVER

Is hay fever an allergy?
Hay fever is usually caused by an allergy to pollen. If problems are experienced, do not ignore them. If the condition is left untreated many other problems may result, as is clearly indicated in my book *Asthma and Bronchitis.*

If hay fever is suspected, start taking Pollinosan towards the end of March (15 drops twice daily). Also take some Echinaforce and Urticalcin. General dietary advice would be to reduce the intake of salt and dairy produce and to take plenty of honey.

What can I take for hay fever?
Follow the advice given in the answer to the previous question. You may consider rounding off the treatment by taking three garlic capsules each night before going to bed.

Could you please advise me on effective treatment methods for hay fever? All members of my family suffer badly.

If all the family suffers, you do indeed have a problem. The general treatment guidelines mentioned above still apply, and I would suggest that you also give your family Imuno-Strength to help boost the immune system. Preferably, however, consult a practitioner for individual advice.

HEADACHES

I feel as if I am never free of a headache. What can I do?

My first advice is never to ignore it. It should be understood that a headache is like an alarm signal. Somewhere in the body something is wrong, and this must be investigated. The root of the problem may be as diverse as stress or a disorder of the liver or gallbladder, and therefore the answer will not be found by taking a few painkillers. This course of action does not eliminate the root of the problem.

If you have the occasional headache, you may be advised to take the natural remedy Petaforce, but any frequent and recurring headache requires more attention. For general advice read my book *Migraine and Epilepsy*.

I have been suffering with headaches, which I get right across my forehead. It is not actually migraine, but my wife thinks that it may be a form of migraine or tension headache. I admit that I am under pressure at present because my company has decided to relocate me. I wonder if you could suggest a form of screening so that the cause of the problem may be discovered, and I would also like to know about any treatment.

Your wife may well be correct in her assumption that this condition is caused by stress. Even so, you do not want to have to live with it. Screening is difficult and you may like to use an individual kind of elimination process. In the meantime, I suggest that you use Neuroforce and *Loranthus*.

I get bad headaches and sickness which last for several days. It starts with a weak back – just below the shoulder blades – and even after the headache and sickness has gone, I feel an imbalance in the spine. Can you offer any advice?

From your brief description, I have no hesitation in stating that the answer to your problems lies in osteopathic treatment. I am sure that with some manipulation and soft-tissue massage your problems can be overcome.

My son has had an almost continuous headache for 5–6 months. He has had two brain scans which have revealed nothing. He describes it as if hot water is being poured on his head and he also gets pins and needles which continues down his arms. He is a hod carrier and admits that when he sits down and relaxes the pains ease. He has tried all kinds of tablets, but nothing has been effective. Do you have any suggestions?

What is sometimes overlooked is that such a condition can be the symptom of a sinus infection. Tell your son to have this possibility checked. On the whole, I would suggest acupuncture treatment and some homoeopathic remedies, e.g. *Spigelia 6x* or *Nat. mur. 6x.*

How does one find relief for severe headache pains at the back of the head, probably caused by tension, without taking drugs?

I would be most surprised if these pains could not be overcome by soft-tissue manipulation. Also, of course, examine your life style and see if it is possible to reduce the stress factor.

I suffer from a one-sided headache with occasional flashing lights and stiffness of the neck. I only sleep for a few hours each night. I have heard your suggestions for relaxation exercises to promote sleep. Is there anything else that could be beneficial?

The exercise you refer to is the 'Hara' breathing method described in my book *Stress and Nervous Disorders.* Your condition appears to be a migraine-type headache and therefore you could also try taking 15 drops of *Loranthus* twice daily and Dr Vogel's Migraine Formula (Formula MGR417).

My headaches are accompanied by light-headedness, although I never actually faint; nausea, but I am never actually sick; palpitations; a shaky feeling when I allow

things to get on top of me; lethargy; falling asleep when I take the weight off my feet; waking up after a full night's sleep, still not feeling refreshed; forgetfulness; swollen legs, mostly at night; and pains in the neck and jaw, similar to those from swollen glands. These are my symptoms, which come and go without a pattern. The problems have developed ever since the birth of my son in 1978 and the hospital's verdict is that I am healthy, although possibly suffering from stress. The latest advice is that if laser treatment does not provide any improvement psychiatric help should be considered. I do not want to go along this road, but I feel helpless.

Your detailed description of your symptoms reminds me of one of my patients. She made a full recovery which was largely based on two remedies: *Centaurium* (15 drops, twice daily) and *Nux vomica 6x*.

HEART PROBLEMS

Is there anything that can be safely taken in order to generally strengthen the heart?

Fortunately, thanks to Mother Nature, there are several remedies to choose from: Hawthorne (Crataegus) and Cardiaforce. These three remedies can be safely used to strengthen the heart and encourage it to perform its vital task.

After a stress test it showed that one day I might need by-pass surgery. Can I do anything to avoid this? If not, what do you suggest should be done to aid recovery?

I would suggest a combination of simple, gentle exercise and the remedy *Ginkgo biloba* to improve the circulation and strengthen the heart. After a by-pass operation you can help your condition significantly by concentrating on strengthening the immune system. Follow a sensible diet, use Imuno-Strength, Crataegus and a low dose of vitamin E.

My husband has recently had a by-pass operation and is slowly recovering. Could you please advise him on diet etc.?

Your husband's condition will be greatly helped by a low-fat diet. For additional advice please read my book *Heart and Blood Circulatory Problems*.

What do you think about taking a vitamin and mineral supplement to strengthen the heart after by-pass surgery? How does one overcome the fatigue problems?
A multivitamin preparation such as Health Insurance Plus will be helpful for fatigue as well as general condition-building.

What about heart flutters? Are these dangerous, because they always frighten me when they occur?
If this happens repeatedly you must go to your doctor. However, heart flutters probably occur more often than we realise. Natural remedies for this occurrence are Cardiaforce or *Melissa off.*, while homoeopathic remedies offer the following choice: *Lycopus viz. 2x, Nat. mur. 6x* or *Belladonna*.

Can you advise any general alternative remedies which can safely be taken alongside medicine prescribed by my doctor?
Crataegus, Auroforce and *Valeriana off.* are all remedies that can safely be used.

Would you prescribe Valerian for people with heart problems? Also, is it true that Valerian or Dormeasan cause a hangover effect?
There is no danger involved if Valerian is used sensibly. With regard to your second question, you may rest assured that I have never heard that either Valerian nor Dormeasan causes a hangover effect.

What about heartburn – is it dangerous?
No, fortunately it is not dangerous, or the majority of people would live in fear. However, whilst it is not dangerous, it is definitely uncomfortable. Generally, heartburn is caused by digestive disorders or because of incorrect eating habits, i.e irregular meals, meals eaten too quickly or a poor diet.

HIATUS HERNIA

I have great problems with hiatus hernia. Can you explain this condition and advise me on its treatment?

A hiatus hernia is the weakening of the tissue around the hole, or hiatus in the diaphragm through which the oesophagus descends into the stomach, sometimes causing exertion, pressure or even a small hairline crack. Sometimes it causes an unpleasantly full and burning sensation. I believe that most cases of hiatus hernia are brought on by people eating too much at one time and eating their food too quickly. For people with this condition the best advice is that six small meals a day are much better than three large meals. Always chew your food very thoroughly. In order to strengthen the tissue, take 15 drops of *Galeopsis* twice daily.

What can one do to avoid hiatus hernia pains?
Always eat your food slowly and do not over-eat. When chewing your food give the saliva a chance to mix properly with the food as this allows the digestive and gastric juices to do their job. It is also worth knowing that a good osteopath or chiropractor should be able to adjust the hiatus.

I have heard that it is possible to adjust a hiatus hernia. Can you tell me if that is true and how is this done?
In my time I have saved many patients from surgery by adjusting the hiatus using a special manipulative technique. Anyone with problems of this nature should seek the advice of a well-qualified osteopath.

Can a hiatus hernia be treated with herbal remedies?
Taking 15 drops of the remedy *Centaurium* twice a day in a little water is helpful.

HYPERACTIVITY

How should a hyperactive child be treated?
The child should first of all be checked for allergies. In many cases I have diagnosed an allergy to sugar in such children. Once an allergy has been pinpointed – sometimes through an elimination process – the treatment is usually self-explanatory.

Can hyperactivity in children be overcome by a change in diet?
This is often the case and for more detailed information I would suggest that you read Chapter 9 of my book *Viruses, Allergies and the Immune System*.

In the case of hyperactive children is it just a case of cutting out additives or is there a more positive therapy?
As I have already stated above, in most cases it is the sugar in sweets and soft drinks that is at fault. However, artificial additives are also often a factor in hyperactivity.

Could you please advise me on homoeopathic treatment and diet for hyperactivity in young children.
All kinds of allergies may be to blame, but sugar is the most common one. A hyperactive child usually reacts very well if given Oil of Evening Primrose, *Avena sativa* or Neuroforce.

I

IMPOTENCE

Can you make any recommendations on how to overcome impotence?
There are various homoeopathic remedies that can be used, e.g. *Acid phos. 3x, Acid picriam 6x, Sabal serr. 2x* and *Lycopodus clav 6x*. Also, take 500 IU of vitamin E and some wheatgerm oil twice daily. More advice on specific male problems can be found under the heading 'Prostate problems' on pages 207-9.

For the last eight years I have been impotent. What is your advice?
Try Masculex together with extra vitamin C.

IMMUNE SYSTEM

I so often read about the immune system and the auto-immune system. How does it work?
I wonder if you realise how difficult it is to find a straightforward answer to your question. The medical profession has a widely varying stance on this subject, but the one thing that all practitioners agree upon is that there is still much to learn on this subject. I have tried to shed some light on this aspect of health in my book *Viruses, Allergies and the Immune System*. All practitioners fortunately agree that our immune system thrives on wholesome food and that the diet should contain plenty of fresh fruit, vegetables and nuts. I always stress the importance of 'fresh', because a tin of tomato soup that bears no resemblance to tomatoes (except the colour) does not contain much goodness for the body.

My general advice would be to ensure that the diet contains ample vitamin C or else take a supplement. Imuno-Strength is also an excellent supplementary remedy.

What are auto-immune diseases and what is the most vulnerable category?

For your information here follows a list of auto-immune problems and the most vulnerable target areas (in italics):

Addison's disease – *adrenal gland*
Auto-immune haemolytic anaemia – *red blood cell membrane proteins*
Crohn's disease – *gut*
Goodpasture's syndrome – *kidneys and lungs*
Graves' disease – *thyroid*
Hashimoto's thyroiditis – *thyroid*
Idiopathic thrombocytopenic purpura – *platelets*
Insulin-dependent Diabetes mellitus – *pancreatic beta cells*
Multiple sclerosis – *brain and spinal cord*
Myasthenia gravis – *nerve/muscle synapses*
Pemphigus vulgaris – *skin*
Pernicious anaemia – *gastric parietal cells*
Poststreptococcal glomerulonephritis – *kidneys*
Psoriasis – *skin*
Rheumatoid arthritis – *connective tissue*
Scleroderma – *heart, lungs, gut, kidneys*
Sjögren's syndrome – *liver, kidneys, brain, thyroid, salivary gland*
Spontaneous infertility – *sperm*
Systematic lupus erythematosus – *DNA, platelets, other tissues*

Could you give us some simple and practical advice on how to improve our immune system?

First and foremost adopt a well-balanced diet, combined with a sensible exercise programme. For an extra boost Imuno-Strength can be helpful.

Do you believe that *Propolis* can improve the immune system?

Although I have had very encouraging feedback from people who use this food supplement, there is no scientific data to back up this claim.

What is the relationship between the ageing process and the immune system, and can damage to the immune system be reversed?

I am sure that with increasing age the effectiveness of the immune system decreases. To me this indicates that as we get older we should take better care of our health.

For multiple sclerosis sufferers, where the immune system function is lowered, what would be a suitable daily quantity of vitamin C to take?

For MS patients I generally recommend the long-term use of at least 2 g of vitamin C daily.

INDIGESTION

What can one do about indigestion?

Indigestion is always a signal that somewhere in the body something is wrong. The problem need not always be serious, but all the same indigestion may be a symptom of an ulcer, colitis, diverticulitis or a similar disorder. If you experience problems, always bear in mind the following rules to avoid indigestion and heartburn:

1. Eat a well-balanced diet that includes fresh fruit, vegetables, and wholegrain breads and cereals. Avoid greasy foods.
2. Eat slowly. Relax for thirty minutes after meals (but do not lie down).
3. Exercise regularly.
4. If you are lactose-intolerant, eliminate milk and milk products from your diet.
5. Do not skip meals, which allows acid to build up in your stomach.
6. Do not pacify your hunger with coffee, which increases the level of stomach acid.
7. If you drink alcohol, do so only with meals or on a full stomach, so the alcohol will not irritate the stomach lining.
8. Do not take aspirin for a hangover. It can further irritate a stomach already irritated by alcohol.
9. Avoid smoking, which decreases the stomach's natural bicarbonate, an acid buffer.

10. Stimulate saliva by chewing gum, sucking on lozenges, or sipping herbal tea. Swallowing and saliva normally wash any residual acid out of the oesophagus back into the stomach.

My husband has problems with his stomach every time he eats.

It is likely that he eats his meals too quickly. Eating meals slowly is very important, because eating quickly often results in an uncomfortable feeling of fullness. Chew the food well so that the saliva can mix with the food, allowing the body to digest it properly. It is helpful to take an enzyme supplement, e.g. Pancreatin, or the herbal remedy *Centaurium*.

What is the best way to balance a diet of fresh fruit and vegetables to avoid making one's bowel movements too frequent?

Always eat fruit and vegetables separately, with at least twenty-minute intervals between meals or snacks. Also remember that there are two fruits, the so-called 'jealous fruits', that should never be eaten together, i.e. melon and banana.

What can I do to avoid severe wind and nausea? These symptoms often cause me to go off food altogether.

Eat your food slowly and take the remedy *Nux vomica*.

I have indigestion and a duodenal ulcer. What is your advice?

First of all I would suggest that you read my book *Stomach and Bowel Disorders* for general dietary advice. Take ten drops of Petaforce together with four Gastronol tablets twice daily.

Is there any recommended treatment for colitis and hiatus hernia?

Hiatus hernia can cause very persistent indigestion, but remember that an osteopath can help here by manipulation. For the colitis problems I would refer you to my book *Stomach and Bowel Disorders*. Always check that your diet is not at fault and take some herbal remedies to help the situation.

What can help a coated tongue and indigestion with wind and flatulence?

Please try the remedy Boldocynara (ten drops after meals twice daily), as this often helps in such circumstances. With regard to your coated tongue, please make an appointment with a qualified naturopathic practitioner or acupuncturist for an accurate diagnosis.

If you feel that you want to cleanse the digestive system, how do you go about it?

A safe and very effective cleansing treatment programme is Dr Vogel's Detox Box Programme. I do this myself every spring and autumn with very positive results.

Since an operation in January 1985 I have suffered from wind in my bowels which I cannot get rid of. I have tried traditional medication without effect.

Flatulence and wind is not an unusual after-effect of an operation. However, it is unusual for it to persist as long as you describe. Every night before going to bed take three 500 mg capsules of Oil of Evening Primrose. Another good remedy to use under these circumstances is DGL from Enzymatic Therapy.

I suffer from stomach problems brought on by stress. These display themselves through flatulence, stomach cramps and diarrhoea. Do you have any suggestions?

To avoid the feelings of flatulence follow the low-stress diet described in my book *Stress and Nervous Disorders*. With regard to the cramp and diarrhoea, take five drops of Arabiaforce twice daily, but remember that this will only be effective if taken in conjunction with the correct diet.

How would you advise a person who suffers from pancreatitis?

Good specific and general advice can be found in my book *Stomach and Bowel Disorders*.

What would you suggest for colitis?

Of prime importance is a well-balanced diet, examples of which can be found in my book *Stomach and Bowel Disorders*. This measure should be backed up with the homoeopathic remedy *Tuberculinum 30*.

I am bothered with too much acid in the stomach.

You will benefit greatly from the Bioforce remedies *Centaurium* and Gastronol.

Almost two years ago my daughter was diagnosed as having Crohn's disease, when she was 15 years old. She was treated in hospital with cortisone and other drugs and is still on a maintenance dose of Asacol. I am interested in your opinion of a natural form of therapy for this illness.

It would be of great help if you read my book *Stomach and Bowel Disorders*, which contains much general and specific advice. I would also recommend that the homoeopathic remedy *Tuberculinum* is necessary for your daughter.

What diet would you recommend for someone recovering from an operation for *Crohn's disease?*

All dietary information is contained in detail in my book *Stomach and Bowel Disorders*.

How would you treat severe attacks of gastritis?

There are two kinds of gastritis: acute and chronic. Both complaints are due to inflammation of the stomach lining, sometimes accompanied by constipation. In many cases a period of fasting is helpful in conjunction with the remedies prescribed by your practitioner. More detailed information on the treatment of this disorder can be found in my book *Stomach and Bowel Disorders*.

I am often troubled with a 'burning' feeling – mostly on the right side of the stomach. I have a hiatus hernia and would like to know if this could be the cause?

This problem should be investigated, because this need not necessarily be the case. However, if the hiatus hernia is inflamed this can be greatly helped by manipulation and the remedy *Galeopsis*.

My daughter suffers from ulcerative colitis (inflamed intestines) and has been told that she will have to take steroids for the rest of her life. Is there a homoeopathic remedy you could suggest?

This is a very unpleasant condition which certainly requires close medical supervision. However, diet is again very important in such cases. My advice would be to avoid pork in any shape or form, citrus fruits, spices, nicotine, alcohol, salt and sugar. There are definitely herbal remedies available that could help your daughter, but in order to prescribe these I would have to see the patient in person. Suggest that she finds herself a qualified alternative practitioner who will advise her.

Can you suggest anything that would be good for gastritis? I have recently returned from hospital and still feel nauseated, weak and prone to fainting.

To overcome the nauseous and weak feeling there are various remedies you could try e.g. Gastronol, *Centaurium* and MegaZyme. The latter is a broad-based spectrum supplement that may help to supplement the body's own digestive enzymes. MegaZyme contains vegetable-origin digestive enzymes, with the emphasis on those that digest a wide range of the complex protein foods such as eggs, cheese, steak, fish, nuts and cereals. MegaZyme is unique, because all the enzymes are acid-stable and are able to retain their digestive capabilities over a wide range of pH variances. They are combined with the herbs peppermint and gentian, which have traditionally been used to help maintain a good digestion.

I have digestive problems and the doctor is sending me for a scan in the belief that the cause could be my gallbladder. Is it still safe for me to take codliver oil?

If there is any doubt as to the correct diagnosis I would forget about the codliver oil for the moment, because this could aggravate the condition if the gallbladder is at the root of the problems. You would be wise to wait for the outcome of the tests.

I am 50 years of age and have three active duodenal ulcers. Is there a natural remedy for me?

You can safely use the two remedies Gastronol and *Centaurium* combined.

I suffer badly from an acid stomach and have just started drinking bottled spring water because I have heard that this may help. Is this true?

Drinking plenty of water is always good for an acid stomach. However, I do not know what variety of bottled water you use, but remember that it is best to drink still water. Sometimes when people with your condition drink fizzy water the reactions may be more severe.

What can be done for someone with a history of colitis, who has recently developed arthritis and is at present in hospital

with severe anaemia? Also, can you tell me if these conditions may be connected?

One thing is certain, all three problems require treatment. It is possible that they are interlinked and therefore the treatment can overlap from one condition to another. There are some good remedies that may be taken, but this should always be done under the supervision of a qualified practitioner. Unfortunately, because lack of detail, I cannot give you more specific advice, but must ask you to seek the advice of a reliable practitioner.

Is there an alternative treatment method for stomach ulcers?

I could reply to this question in a number of ways, depending upon the condition of the person concerned. For both general and more detailed advice I suggest that you read my book *Stomach and Bowel Disorders*.

I suffer from severe diverticulitis and would like any suggestions for a homoeopathic remedy.

If you were my patient, depending on the findings of my examination, I would recommend one or more of the following homoeopathic remedies: *Lycopodium, Ignatia, Dioscorea* and sometimes *Thuja*.

My mother has been ill for five years with digestive problems. She wonders if it is due to a fungal disease in the digestive system. She has problems digesting food although she has a good diet. She is capable of putting on weight overnight and of losing it the next night. She also has dark circles under her eyes. Can you advise her?

Your mother should be examined thoroughly because there are many external indications and a practitioner may well diagnose her as suffering from *Candida albicans*, which is a yeast parasite. My advice is to seek the help of a good practitioner.

What treatment and dietary changes do you recommend for a duodenal ulcer?

Specific dietary advice can be found in my book *Stomach and Bowel Disorders*, which also contains suggestions on suitable remedies for ulcer conditions.

Is diverticulitis curable and is there a specific diet one should follow?

Diverticulitis may not be curable in the true sense of the word, but it is definitely controllable! Guidelines for special diets that help to keep this condition under control, together with advice on suitable remedies can be found in my book *Stomach and Bowel Disorders*.

Sometimes people find difficulty in changing over to a wholefood diet – particularly elderly people. They experience indigestion and flatulence. Can you give advice on how to cope with this? Should they change over gradually? Should they study particular combinations of foods, etc.?
Sometimes food-combining is needed and for specific advice here I would recommend that you read my book *Nature's Gift of Food*. Your suggestion to effect any change in the diet gradually shows a sensible approach.

INFECTIONS

Why is there so much talk of infections nowadays and why do we constantly hear about new ones?
My theory is that because of adverse changes to the environment our immune system is under more stress than at any time previously. This renders us more vulnerable to passing infections, which sometimes can develop into new strains. Always remember that prevention is better than cure and for people who are especially vulnerable I am likely to prescribe Echinaforce, vitamin C and Imuno-Strength, in order to give them the added protection required.

My grandson is five years old and suffering from pneumonia. He is now on penicillin medication, but I wonder if there is a homoeopathic remedy that might have been useful?
In many cases I have been able to help patients suffering from such conditions with Echinaforce, which is the most marvellous natural antibiotic.

It is one year now since I had pneumonia, and yet I still experience recurring low fevers, night sweats and fatigue. As I do not use dairy foods, I wonder if this could be because of low calcium?

Pneumonia is an inflammation of the lungs caused by colds or influenza, although it can also be a viral infection. Take plenty of vitamin C – at such times up to 4 g daily may be allowed – and Echinaforce. You are correct in your assumption that sometimes a low calcium level may have a bearing on the situation and I would therefore also suggest that you take four tablets of Urticalcin twice daily.

I have had a respiratory infection for three years and for the last two years I have been continuously on antibiotics. If I do not take these tablets I get pneumonia, but on the other hand the penicillin makes me hoarse, gives me bronchial spasms so that I cannot lie down and, furthermore, makes my joints swell. Is there an alternative?
Take 20 drops of Echinaforce twice daily and to help strengthen the immune system take one Imuno-Strength tablet three times daily.

A little while ago my mother had an accident in which she hurt her leg. That leg has now become ulcerated and infected. It is painful to the touch. Is there anything she can take for this?
Your mother will benefit greatly if she takes the following:

1. Ten drops of *Hamamelis virg.* (witch hazel) twice before meals.
2. Ten drops of Petaforce, twice daily after meals.
3. Up to 1,000 IU vitamin E daily.

My granddaughter is 17 years old and just recovering from glandular fever. Can you suggest something to boost her immune system to prevent a recurrence?
Advise her to take one tablet of Imuno-Strength twice daily. This will help her to build up her reserves.

Can you advise me on how to avoid or treat *Herpes simplex* (cold sores)?
Take one tablet of Viraplex together with two tablets of Health Insurance Plus, both twice daily.

What would you give for a persistent bad cough?
Take ten drops of *Lachesis 8x.* twice daily. Gargle with diluted Molkosan

and, twice daily, take 20 drops of Echinaforce. This will help you to eliminate the infection.

What do you recommend for fungal infections affecting the feet?

Take 20 drops of Echinaforce twice daily. For external treatment I would recommend dabbing the nails daily with *Spilanthes*, which is an excellent remedy specifically for fungal infections.

My husband has *Otitis media* ever since going swimming 15 years ago in Yugoslavia. All this time he has been on drugs to contain this condition but has now discovered that these tablets affect his hearing. Is there a homoeopathic alternative?

This condition is caused by germs spreading in the Eustachian tube, which connects the nose to the throat. I would imagine that your husband has avoided swimming ever since, which is a very sensible precaution. For his deafness I would suggest supplementary zinc and selenium along with the homoeopathic remedy *Belladonna 30x* and the herbal remedy *Plantago majalis*.

Can you recommend a single homoeopathic remedy that can be used for infections?

In the homoeopathic field I mostly recommend *Lachesis 8x*, often backed up with Echinaforce. To my mind the latter is the most effective natural antibiotic.

My daughter has had glandular fever for two months now. Her GP said just to give it time. Have you any suggestions?

I must stress that glandular fever should never be ignored, because there are many ME patients nowadays who are suffering because they under-estimated an attack of glandular fever and failed to obtain reliable medical advice. Take Echinaforce and Kelpasan, and to boost the immune system follow Dr Vogel's Detox Box Programme.

Is there any homoeopathic cure for an infection in the upper jaw? I have had a cyst removed and now there is some infection. Antibiotics do not work.

Take ten drops of *Lachesis 8x* twice daily before meals and also 20 drops of

Echinaforce twice daily. Gently dab *Propolis* ointment onto the gums – morning and night.

My 40-year-old sister had meningitis last summer, which resulted in a total loss of hearing in one ear and partial deafness in the other ear. At a recent hearing test it was discovered that some hearing is returning to the ear in which she was totally deaf. Is there anything she could take to help her hearing to return?
Meningitis is a viral or bacterial infection of the delicate membranes – the so-called meninges – surrounding the brain. In your sister's case the hearing ability has been affected and I would advise her to take *Arnica 3x* and *Bryonia 30x*. Tell your sister that acupuncture can often bring about the desired improvement.

INFERTILITY

Can anything be done for infertility?
I am pleased to say that I have helped a number of patients with this unfortunate problem. However, medical checks for ovulation and sperm count, etc. must take place to ascertain that there are no medical causes for this condition to persist. A personal consultation is essential, as the condition may be dependent upon a large variety of seemingly unrelated factors.

My husband and I have been trying for a family for over two years now. Medical tests have shown that our fertility is not in doubt, but still nothing has happened. Can you make any suggestions to improve our chances?
There are various ways of approaching your request. Certainly as far as remedies are concerned I would supplement your vitamin and mineral intake and specifically advise you to consider taking a larger than usual dosage of vitamin E and calcium. Seek the help of a reliable osteopath, because there may be some pressure on the womb, not forgetting that ovarian treatment may also be required.

Are there any herbs or other products which can aid a male with a low sperm count who wishes to father children?
The remedy Masculex has produced some very encouraging results.

INFLUENZA

What can one do about an attack of flu?

Do not ever suppress a bout of flu, but let it run its course and help the system to overcome it. My grandmother – a wise lady with a great deal of knowledge on naturopathic medicine – used to say: 'Give me a flu and I can treat all ills.' By using water-treatment methods as advised in my book *Water – Healer or Poison?* the healing crisis can be brought to a head, to be followed by a quick recovery. By suppressing illnesses such as flu, colds and infections many people have turned into chronic invalids.

Naturopathy, once thought to be a form of crankiness, has now proved itself to be an effective, scientific and highly beneficial form of therapy, and in many European countries it is now offered on a par with allopathic medicine.

The basic principle of naturopathy is the *Vis Medicatrix Naturae* – that it is the inherent Life Force which heals. This force is stimulated by those factors which normally promote health and it is suppressed by excesses and deficiencies. The *materia medica* is fasting, following the correct diet, restoration of structural integrity (osteopathy), hydrotherapy, heliotherapy (sunlight), deep-breathing, appropriate exercise, optimum relaxation and sleep and the removal of noxious influences. Water has been used extensively and has been found to be almost miraculous in its therapeutic action. Many diseases respond so well to therapeutic fasting that the early naturopaths regarded it as a panacea.

What natural remedies can one use to prevent colds and flu?

Due to cold, stress and inadequate nutrition our immune system becomes less effective and therefore more vulnerable. If this is the case it can be helped by avoiding sugar and sugary foods. Drink plenty of still mineral water and herbal tea, and eat light meals. Take up to 3–4 g of vitamin C per day and also 15 drops of Echinaforce three times daily. A multivitamin preparation and supplementary zinc and garlic are also advisable.

INSOMNIA AND SLEEP DISORDERS

How many hours sleep should one have?

The average person requires some 7–8 hours of sleep per night and, although it is considered an old wives' tale, the hours of sleep before midnight are the most beneficial. Bear in mind that our lymphatic system replenishes itself best during sleep.

My husband is a great worrier and has insomnia and is often affected by nightmares. Do you have any advice for curing insomnia?

Suggest to your husband that he takes a brisk walk late in the evening, followed by a warm drink of *Melissa* and honey together with 30 drops of Dormeasan before retiring to bed. This often works well, but if there is still no improvement he may be advised to undergo some acupuncture treatment.

How does one close one's mind to concerns and worries in order to sleep?

Practise relaxation exercises, such as listening to a tape of soothing music, or read up on some meditating techniques.

My husband is 62 years old and we would like your advice on how to help him establish a regular sleeping pattern. He sleeps, but not for long enough and not during the acceptable night time hours.

Often this is a matter of habit. With perseverance your husband should be able to change the habit back to taking his sleep during the acceptable hours, i.e. night-time.

I suffer from periodic bouts of insomnia and Valerian is not effective.

Although Valerian is a very useful medication, I know that it is not always effective. I would suggest that you try Dormeasan or Jayvee tablets. Remember that routine is very important for a regular sleeping pattern.

What dosage of Valerian is required for an adult who suffers from insomnia?

In most cases about 20 drops taken half an hour before going to bed is effective.

Can one sleep for too long, i.e. is 12 hours too much?

Some people require more sleep than others, although twelve hours a night does seem a long time for an adult. The average is approximately 7–8 hours. If you cannot manage with less than 12 hours you may wish to consider having a medical check-up.

What can one do about sleeping disorders (trouble falling asleep and staying awake)?

This is possibly a case of narcolepsy, a condition that unfortunately, is not yet fully understood but is frequently diagnosed in ME sufferers. Drowsiness is generally due to an excess of vitamin D. However, if it is caused by narcolepsy, there are many good remedies available and I would suggest that you seek individual advice from a qualified practitioner.

Since my early twenties I have suffered from narcolepsy (falling asleep). I was given Benzedrine, which is now no longer available. Is there anything I can take to help?

There is a homoeopathic remedy called *Cerebrum* which is often helpful for the condition you describe. You could also try an enzyme product called Escalation Formula, which has been used with very good results.

Can you advise on sleeping problems? I regularly wake up several times during the night especially at 3.00 a.m.

This is often due to habitual circumstances, e.g. requiring the use of the toilet at about that time of the night. Study the Hara breathing method as outlined in my book *Stress and Nervous Disorders*.

Can you give some practical methods or advice on curing insomnia? Although I do some yoga exercises to relax me before going to bed, I still find it difficult to fall asleep.

As well as relaxation exercises you may like to try some meditation. Take a brisk walk in the fresh air during the latter part of the evening and try taking 30 drops of Dormeasan half an hour before going to bed.

I would like to know if anything can be done for ongoing insomnia. I have had these problems for at least 25 years.

Take 30 drops of Dormeasan, half an hour before going to bed, together with a relaxing hot drink. A brisk walk in the evening will also help. Remember that you will have to grow out of your current sleeping pattern and slowly develop a new one.

IRRITABLE BOWEL SYNDROME

There is so much mention of irritable bowel syndrome today. Could you please tell me what causes this condition?
The common denominators that bring about this condition are mainly stress, coffee, alcohol and spices. The better you are able to relax the less likely you are to suffer from this condition. A very good remedy is *Centaurium* (15 drops, twice daily before meals). A recently rediscovered remedy is peppermint oil. For centuries this has been used as an aid to maintaining normal digestion. It is not by chance that mints are often eaten after meals and this tradition has developed because people appreciate the warm comfortable feeling that these sweets induce.

However, peppermint oil capsules should not be confused with sweets. Each capsule of Nature's Best's Peppermint Oil provides a potent 50 mg of peppermint oil, which is many times stronger than even the hottest mint. Peppermint oil is distilled from the plant's leaves and because this precious essential oil is quite volatile it is believed that the only way to prevent it evaporating is to encapsulate it in a base of sunflower oil. When the capsule releases the peppermint oil in the stomach it helps to regulate the digestion.

How are intestinal irritations and inflammation diagnosed?
Often the patient will complain of irregular bowel movements, combined with itching of the skin, although they rarely realise there may be a link between the two symptoms. Tests can be done and it is surprising how useful an iridology test is in such circumstances. Many problems become apparent during an iridology test because the eyes provide us with a finely tuned analysis of the patient's biochemistry and of emotional and circumstantial factors which are hard to determine by any other method. Iridology is the science of analysing the delicate structures of the iris of the eye. Under magnification using a biomicroscope, the iris reveals itself as a world of minute details – a complete map that represents a communication system capable of handling an amazing quantity of information.

The iris is an extension of the brain and is prolifically endowed with hundreds of thousands of nerve endings, microscopic blood vessels, muscles and other tissues. Each iris is connected to every organ and tissue of the body via the brain and nervous system. The nerve fibres receive their impulses by way of their connection to the optic nerve, optic thalamus and spinal cord. They are formed embryologically from mesoderm and neuroectoderm tissues, and both the sympathetic and parasympathetic nervous systems are present in the iris. In this way, Nature has provided us with a miniature television screen showing the most remote parts of the body, which normally cannot be seen by conventional diagnostic methods, by way of nerve reflex responses.

I have had an irritable colon for some years. I am trying to withdraw from tranquillisers, but this has made the irritable colon worse. I'd be grateful for your advice.

Tranquillisers keep this condition artificially under control. Remember that a spastic colon condition can be effectively treated with a well-balanced diet and for advice in this area I would refer you to my book *Stomach and Bowel Disorders*. An excellent remedy to help overcome tranquilliser dependency and at the same time regulate and ease bowel disruptions is Ginsavena (15 drops, twice daily).

Do you have any suggestions please on what I can do for irritable bowel syndrome?

First of all make sure that you are not constipated. If that is the case, use Dr Vogel's Linoforce, which is a gentle yet effective means to regulate the bowel movements. In the case of loose bowel movements take Tormentavena and remember to limit your intake of coffee, alcohol and spices.

Could you please tell me something about irritable bowel syndrome. I am scheduled to see a specialist on this complaint in two months time and I am not looking forward to it.

Take action now! Read my book *Stomach and Bowel Disorders* for general advice and adapt your diet accordingly. Take Peppermint Oil capsules and if the bowel is spastic take 15 drops of Ginsavena twice daily.

What would you suggest for irritable bowel syndrome, most likely induced by constipation?

Many of my patients have successfully controlled this condition by the simple means of chewing half a teaspoon of Linoforce granules twice daily.

What do you think is the cause of an irritable colon and what can be done about it?

This condition is often induced by stress or colon/vegetative neurosis. Sometimes a mucous colitis condition can be at the root of the problem. Much useful advice can be found in my book *Stomach and Bowel Disorders*.

For five years now I have suffered from irritable bowel syndrome and frequently suffer from severe wind spasms. What is your advice?

Pay attention to the general advice given in answer to the previous questions on the same subject. Especially for wind and flatulence I would recommend *Centaurium* (15 drops, twice daily).

J

JAUNDICE

What treatment would you recommend for jaundice?

First, I suggest that you consult your GP in order to determine the cause of your jaundice. Once an accurate diagnosis has been made there are a number of measures you can take. Each day, take Boldocynara and Dr Vogel's Liver and Gall Bladder Formula (Formula LGB). The following homoeopathic remedies are also suitable for the treatment of jaundice: *Lycopodium virg. 2x Bryonia alba 4x, Chelidonium 2x* and *Taraxacum off.*

K

KIDNEY DISORDERS

What general steps can be taken to care for one's kidneys?
The kidneys require frequent cleansing, which can be achieved by drinking plenty of fluid, preferably still mineral water, as fizzy water will be less effective. Also, use salt sparingly because this unnecessarily burdens the kidneys.

I have been told that I have a virus in my kidney and that this is the reason why I appear to be staggering. My eyesight is not very good and I have been advised not to drive a car. My doctor has prescribed steroids and Oil of Evening Primrose. This condition has now been ongoing for nine weeks and I would be grateful for your advice.
Drink plenty of water to cleanse your kidneys as well as you can. Twice a day before meals take 20 drops of Echinaforce and after meals take 15 drops of Nephrosolid in a cup of Golden Grass Tea, also twice daily.

Can very strong smelling urine be overcome by herbal medication, and please tell me if this is a sign of kidney trouble?
Your suspicion of kidney problems is a possibility, but instead of fearing the worst, it would be much better if you had your urine checked. For your kidneys, drink plenty of water and herbal teas, e.g. camomile tea, Jan de Vries Health Tea, or Golden Grass Tea.

Is it possible for a severe throat infection to leave a weakness in the left kidney?
Yes, this is possible. It depends on how this infection has travelled through the body, but in such cases the kidneys can sometimes become involved. Follow the advice given in answer to the previous question.

My granddaughter is three years old and has been diagnosed as having too much albumen in the blood stream resulting in a kidney infection. Her little body is swollen due to the kidneys not functioning correctly and she has gained 2 kg with body fluid. The doctor has put the child on cortisone for about four weeks. What can she be given after the cortisone treatment is finished? Also, will she suffer any lasting effects and is it possible that the problems may recur? Finally, what could have caused this condition in the first place?

It is very difficult to accurately state what the cause of this condition may have been, because it could have been triggered by an infection or a blood disorder. In such cases, however, cortisone is often prescribed. Alternatively, I would prescribe five drops of Petaforce and five drops of Nephrosolid, both twice daily.

What do you know about the Manehurrian mushroom, Kombucha or Karsagak tea, which is fermented with black tea and brown sugar? Is it helpful for the kidneys?

I have heard that in some countries this is promoted as a way of cleansing the kidneys, but personally I have never come across any practitioner who used this combination and therefore have no exact details as to its effectiveness.

I have a considerable problem with water retention, even though I am on a salt-free diet. I swell up immediately if I eat any salt at all. Can you please advise me?

Indeed, you should continue to follow a salt-free diet and, contrary to what many people believe, you should drink plenty of fluids, preferably water, because water is the best diuretic. Also eat plenty of celeriac and celery.

I have only one kidney and would be pleased to learn what preventive healthcare you would advise.

Take good care of your one kidney and you should be able to cope without any major problems. Drink plenty of fluids, including vegetable juices and herbal teas, and from time to time take a course of Nephrosolid.

Can you give me some advice for my husband? He has had problems with one kidney for 16 years now. He has been to

see a number of doctors, but they cannot find or confirm anything. Recently, a reflexologist confirmed a problem with his kidney and said that it is building up gravel or stones. He has quite painful spasmodic pains in his side.

Such conditions are often accurately diagnosed during reflexology treatment and therefore I suspect that the diagnosis is correct. Encourage your husband to follow a salt-free diet and complement this with ten drops of Nephrosolid in a cup of Golden Grass Tea twice daily. To avoid the build up of gravel or stones I would suggest Tarxacum officinalis twice daily 15 drops.

Can you please advise me on how to cleanse the kidneys in the case of an oedema?

Drink plenty of fluids and every day take 15 drops of Nephrosolid in a cup of Kidney Tea.

How are kidney stones formed and, more importantly, how can they be avoided?

Kidney stones or renal calculi are hard pieces of calcium and other salts, which accumulate in the larger urine-collecting ducts. Homoeopathic medicine is often helpful, e.g. *Berberis 6x, Cantharis 6x* and *Lycopodium 6x*. Also, take half a teaspoon of glycerine in the morning, and be careful with your vitamin C and calcium intake. Avoid salt or alcohol and reduce the intake of lactose or fructose. Follow a high-fibre diet and try not to become overweight.

I regularly suffer from kidney stones. I have been told that they are made of calcium oxalate and therefore I might have to avoid certain foods.

Kidney stones can cause a lot of misery and pain and the oxalate type of stone has sharp edges and is therefore particularly sore. You should exclude from your diet all chocolate, tea, rhubarb, spinach, broccoli, strawberries, asparagus and tomatoes. Drink at least four pints of still mineral water daily. Take 15 drops of Nephrosolid in some Golden Grass Tea three times daily and every morning take half a teaspoon of glycerine.

What can be done for an oedema which has been brought about by malfunction of the kidneys?

Eat plenty of celery, asparagus and celeriac. There are a number of remedies that are beneficial for such conditions, such as Convascillan, Nephrosolid, Golden Grass Tea and *Solidago.*

L

LIVER DISORDERS

What can be done about a suspected sluggish liver?
Take ten drops of Boldocynara twice daily and pay strict attention to your diet. The dietary guidelines given below are specifically designed for patients with diagnosed or suspected liver problems.

Liver Diet

Recommended foods
Take only vegetables, especially raw. Dress salads with Molkosan (a milk-whey product). Use buttermilk, natural yoghurt (low fat), toasted wholemeal bread, potatoes, Ryvita, natural brown rice, grapefruit, grapes and berries, sunflower or olive oil and honey. Drink herbal teas, apple juice, and blackcurrant juice.

Do not use
Coffee, tea, white sugar or white flour (and products made with them), vinegar, tinned products, fruits other than those indicated above, meat, butter, fried foods, spices, cucumber, cabbage, cauliflower or spinach. No sweets or chocolates.

General advice
Each day eat two plates of grated carrots. Walk for about one hour daily. One day a week should be a fasting day, when only apple juice, camomile tea and carrot juice may be taken. Twice each day spend fifteen minutes on breathing exercises.

Recommended cooking method for whole brown rice
Place the rice in a casserole or pyrex dish and cover with boiling milk or water. Have the oven ready on a high temperature. Cook the rice for only

10–15 minutes before switching off the oven. Keep the rice in the oven for a further 5–6 hours. Chop some vegetables such as parsley, chicory, celery and cress and mix these through the rice together with a little garlic salt. Reheat the rice before serving.

I have to take steroids for hepatitis but they are giving me stomach problems (indigestion, etc.). Is there anything I can take to relieve the stomach pain?

Take ten drops of Petaforce twice daily together with two tablets of *Hepar sulph. D4*. Also eat plenty of artichokes, which are excellent for the liver.

What remedy would you suggest for liver problems?

The best remedy is Boldocynara and I have used this for many years for my patients. Milk thistle extract (Silybum marianum) is also very effective. This plant is found in certain parts of Europe, where it is an established herbal supplement. As with many herbal products its reported properties have recently been verified through scientific research.

Silymarin is the name of the active extract from the fruit and consists of three kinds of flavonoligams. Silymarin has been shown to help maintain the health of the liver; it scavenges free radicals and may help to maintain the rate of cell renewal in the liver.

The liver operates at a high speed, cleansing the blood of the harmful toxins taken in with our food and with the polluted air that we breathe, those produced by bacteria in the gut, and of course toxins such as alcohol that we choose to consume. This detoxifying action exerts a severe toll on cells of the liver and for this reason cell turnover needs to be very fast. Human studies have shown that following oral administration, elements of silymarin stay specifically in the liver (rather than circulating in the blood).

I need help for hepatitis C – a condition of the liver. For your information, I do not drink.

Hepatitis C is a serious condition, but is fortunately rather rare. Medical help is essential for this condition and the following guidelines should be adhered to if alternative treatment is preferred. Take Petaforce (ten drops, twice daily), additional vitamin C and also *Chelidonium*. Most doctors or practitioners are not opposed to combining alternative treatment with allopathic treatment in such cases, but medical supervision is always necessary.

Can someone whose spleen has been removed still keep the liver in order? Does it make a difference?
You may rest assured that with good guidance from a doctor or practitioner the liver can be helped to function correctly, even without the spleen.

Are you in favour of Interferon injections for fatty liver?
Although I have heard of this treatment method, I have not seen any reports on its effectiveness and therefore I cannot make any recommendations as to any possible benefits.

Please could I have your comments on a rare liver disorder – microcystic disease? I have a poor bile flow and stone formation in the liver.
Follow the liver diet as outlined on pages 150-1 and also take Boldocynara each day.

How would you go about removing metal toxicity in the liver and other glands in the system?
In these circumstances the Detox Box Programme is invaluable.

Please explain about liver-cleansing programmes, and certain apple juice and olive oil programmes for this purpose. Also please tell me whether, in your opinion, the emotions are a primary factor with liver congestion?
There are several liver-cleansing programmes and a number of them can be found in my book *Traditional Home and Herbal Remedies*. The apple and olive oil course is also described there. As for the second part of your question: the liver is very much subject to emotions. Stress and emotional strain have an adverse effect on the liver, and a nervous breakdown is often the cause of an impaired liver function. If you consider that 1,200 pints of blood are filtered by the liver during a span of 24 hours, you will realise that it makes good sense to take care of the liver.

LYMPH GLANDS

Is it true that the lymph glands gather a large amount of toxic material in the course of a day?

The lymph glands swell up during infections and this is always an indication that help is necessary. Much waste material causes problems and the lymph glands do a very worthwhile job, especially during the night when we are asleep. This is the time that they set about cleansing the system, and to help them in this work you would be advised to take three capsules of Oil of Evening Primrose at night before going to bed.

M

MENOPAUSE

Is it true that a woman can stay in the 'change of life' for many years?

Indeed, some women do. However, there are many ways to help and get through this period without experiencing too many problems. In fact, some women do not even have the slightest symptoms of the hormonal changes that are taking place in their bodies. Recently there has been much publicity on the subject of HRT preparations, but I am very much in favour of trying alternative ways, such as diet, vitamin supplements, herbal remedies, relaxation and exercise. It is important to maintain a positive outlook and, to that end, it is worthwhile remembering that 'life begins at 50'.

What vitamin supplements would you suggest for women in the menopause?

Many of my female patients in the relevant age group have reported good results after they started to use Gynovite Plus. This is a preparation especially designed for women during and after the menopause. The formula places emphasis on minerals that are essential in the diet for helping to maintain the bone health of menopausal women. Although calcium is important for bone health, it is not over-emphasised in Gynovite. This is because the absorption and metabolism of this mineral is delicately balanced by a system of hormones which controls the calcium level in the body. When blood calcium is low, intestinal absorption of this mineral is increased and renal excretion decreased. Magnesium plays an important part in bone health and too much calcium interferes with the absorption and action of this mineral.

Gynovite contains a high level of magnesium, a mineral that is essential for the well-being of women in the later years of life. An adequate intake of magnesium facilitates calcium absorption and utilisation, thus decreasing the need for a high level of calcium in the supplement. The Women's Nutritional Advisory Service recommend Gynovite as part of a total programme consisting of changes in life style, dietary habits and exercise. The latter is important in the maintenance of bone health, with weight-bearing exercise in particular being believed to reduce the natural slow loss of calcium from bones that is common in post-menopausal women.

I am 49 years old and have been going through the menopause for two years. I have a tremor going through my legs and believe this to be arthritis. What can be done?
First of all make sure that you follow a healthy diet; I would specifically point to the dietary guidelines mentioned in my book *Arthritis, Rheumatism and Psoriasis.* Secondly, the Menopause Formula will help, and Seatone – a mussel extract – is of particular benefit to women in the menopause.

I have been ill for quite a few years, suffering from heavy periods. The medicine prescribed by my doctor made me ill and he told me that the only solution would be a hysterectomy. At that time, I consulted a homoeopathic practitioner, who put me on what he called a 'constitutional remedy'. Since then I have lost some 20 pounds, I feel very much better and have lots of energy. Now I would like to share my experience with other women.
Homoeopathic treatment often works very well, and a constitutional remedy I often prescribe is called *Menosan.* Dr Vogel often recommends the use of Ovasan. Both remedies have had very supportive and encouraging feedback.

I am in the middle of the change of life and suffering from hot flushes, especially at night, with the result that I am not sleeping very well. Can you please help?
The herbal remedy *Salvia* (or sage) is very helpful for hot flushes or night sweats. It is interesting to know the peculiarities of this herb, because when the sun comes out sage specks of 'perspiration' appear on its leaves, more or less like the sudden flushes that befall menopausal women. It is therefore a perfect example of the principle of 'Like cures Like'.

I have had a mastectomy and am now suffering from hot flushes. I was put on HRT patches, which affected me unpleasantly and therefore I have been taken off them. Is there anything else that I can do to prevent these hot flushes?
The experience of hot flushes is not unusual after a mastectomy, because the hormonal system usually becomes imbalanced. The sooner you try to regain this balance the better, and I would suggest that you read my book *Menopause* for further advice.

What is the recommended dosage of *Salvia* for treating a hormone imbalance?
Take 15 drops of *Salvia* twice daily before meals.

Oil of Evening Primrose is renowned for its many healing properties, in particular for its GLA content and help with 'women's problems'. Starflower/borage oil claims to have a higher percentge of GLA, but are its healing properties as good?
I have tried them all with patients and, in my experience, the 'healing properties' as you put it, of Evening Primrose are by far the best.

What would you recommend as a calcium supplement for women in their fifties?
For me there is only one calcium preparation and that is Urticalcin. There are many other calcium preparations on the market, but very few are in a form that can be readily absorbed by the body. When formulating Urticalcin Dr Vogel used homoeopathic calcium and mixed it with an extract from the stinging nettle – *Urtica dioica*. The nettle extract facilitates the absorption of calcium into the blood, reducing the risk of calcium deposits.

Could you recommend a herbal supplement in place of HRT for the menopause? Are borage oil capsules an alternative to Oil of Evening Primrose, or perhaps even better?
For a balanced herbal supplement to replace the use of HRT I would suggest tha vitamin supplement Gynovite. Also consider the use of *Menosan* and Oil of Evening Primrose (three capsules taken last thing at night). As for the second part of your question, in my experience Oil of Evening Primrose is more effective than borage oil.

What do you recommend for severe period pains during early menopause?

From reliable feedback from my patients I can wholeheartedly recommend Optivite, a preparation that has been formulated for menstruating women by a former professor of obstetrics and gynaecology. Optivite is highly recommended as being the best specialist multivitamin and mineral product for women who want to supplement their diet throughout their monthly cycle. This formula has been produced after years of studying hormones and how their production in the body is influenced by vitamins and minerals. It was found that many women were at risk of not obtaining sufficient nutrients from their diets and that the dietary habits of others were actually depleting their nutritional status.

Many women who have found vitamin B_6 to be a useful supplement are pleased to find that the recommended daily intake of Optivite (two tablets) provides 100 mg of this essential nutrient. The vitamin B_6 level separates Optivite from other vitamin nutrient formulas, as does the excellent level of vitamin C, which at two tablets provides 500 mg of this important anti-oxidant.

The results of studies commissioned by the Women's Nutritional Advisory Service have emphasised that Optivite works best as part of a complete health-building programme that includes adequate exercise, effective rest and relaxation and a proper diet that may also include a supplement of Evening Primrose Oil.

What herbal remedies would you recommend for pre-menstrual syndrome during the menopause?

Depending upon the individual circumstances, I would recommend any one or more of the following: *Menosan*, *Pulsatilla*, *Hypericum* or coneflower.

How much and what kind of calcium should a woman in the menopause use?

I would recommend taking five tablets of Urticalcin twice daily.

What do you recommend to prevent bone loss after the menopause?

Take five tablets of Urticalcin twice daily and three capsules of Oil of Evening Primrose last thing at night.

I have heard that ginseng can cause an imbalance in a woman's hormones. Do you think it is OK for women to take ginseng, especially during or after the menopause?
You may rest assured that ginseng will not do any harm if you adhere to the recommended dosage as mentioned on the packaging.

I have fibroid tumours in the uterus. Does Dong Quai help produce more oestrogen, and is it therefore not suitable for the reduction of fibroids? What does help to reduce oestrogen in terms of fibroids?
Very little research has taken place on the herb Dong Quai, but it is recommended as a suitable remedy for the menopausal period. A good remedy is Femtol from Enzymatic Therapy, which can reduce the fibroids, taken together with Petaforce.

As I suffer from fibroids is it safe to take hormone replacement therapy (HRT)? If not, is there an alternative I can take to reduce the hot flushes and sweats?
Hormone replacement therapy is considered to be safe with respect to the presence of fibroids. However, I have come across a few exceptions where the patient was advised to avoid HRT preparations. For alternative methods for dealing with your problem, read my book *Menopause*.

My hormonal balance is biased towards an excess of testosterone (I am female and 39 years old). This causes acne, particularly on my chin. To counteract this I have been prescribed 'Dianette' – an artificial female hormone, taken like the contraceptive pill. Is there any natural remedy which would help me? (I have just discovered that my ovaries are not, and possibly never have been, functioning normally.)
Suitable alternative options are *Ovarium* or Gynovite. For more detailed advice please read my book *Menstrual and Pre-Menstrual Tension*.

What do you think of HRT in the form of patches?
As you must have realised from my answers to earlier questions, I am very much in favour of using natural alternatives.

Can you advise on pre-menstrual tension for a friend who suffers with it very badly, i.e. she experiences depression and

pains and is often tearful? I must add that she is approaching the menopause.

Advise your friend to increase her intake of zinc. As women approach the menopause a shortage of zinc often becomes apparent, which expresses itself through the individual feeling weepy and depressed.

Zinc is a trace mineral that is essential for plants, animals and human beings. It is one of the oldest minerals known to man and is a cofactor to more than 80 enzymes in the body, being involved in hundreds of metabolic pathways. It is only available from the diet and is present in the earth's crust where it is usually found in conjunction with other minerals, such as manganese. The highest concentrations of zinc in the adult body are found in the bones, liver, kidneys, pancreas and muscle tissues. One-fifth of the zinc found in the body is in the skin and zinc is well-known for its role in tissue repair (particularly in relation to the skin). The body's supply of zinc has a rapid turnover rate, which is why it is important to ensure a regular and sufficient intake. Zinc is required for:

- growth, where it is necessary for efficient utilisation of nitrogen and sulphur, both in the production of protein and in the synthesis of DNA, and plays a crucial role in cell repair and metabolism. It is vital that children and adolescents receive enough;

- the transport of carbon dioxide – the waste product of the body's use of oxygen – from working tissues to the lungs. Many of the enzymes it works with are associated with this process;

- its role in the immune system;

- the balance of blood sugar through insulin;

- maintaining a healthy liver, vision, our sense of smell and taste and the digestion of carbohydrates;

- the healthy function of reproductive organs and the prostate glands. It is a component of semen;

- the absorption of other nutrients such as vitamin A and the B-complex vitamins.

According to leading researchers in nutrition, more people find it difficult to obtain enough zinc in their diet than they do any other mineral. Soil deficiencies of zinc have reduced the levels available in vegetables and a further quantity of zinc is removed by food processing. High levels of calcium and phosphates found in vegetables are thought to inhibit the absorption of zinc and intake may be threatened by missing meals or fasting. The most reliable food sources of zinc are oysters, herrings, milk, meat and eggs, since zinc from animal and fish sources is much better absorbed, due to the high cysteine content of animal-derived foods.

Fruit and vegetables are poor sources of zinc and many vegetarians and vegans choose to augment their intake with supplements. The average diet provides approximately 10–15 mg of zinc, of which only 20 per cent is absorbed by the body. Many experts estimate that we need between 15 and 20 mg per day in our diet. Smokers and drinkers, contraceptive pill users, the elderly and athletes (zinc is lost in perspiration) often choose to take extra zinc.

I have heard about preparations that should be taken for hot flushes, but I can only remember that one was Oil of Evening Primrose, together with something else. Can you help?
For hot flushes and night sweats I would recommend *Menosan*, taken in combination with Oil of Evening Primrose.

Is there anything in alternative medicine to help 'flushes and sweats'? I am nearly 60 years of age and just finishing the menopause. Nothing the doctor has given me helps. I have also seen a specialist, who has assured me that the problem has nothing to do with my glands.
Taking into account your age I would suggest that you take additional vitamin C: take one 500 IU capsule twice daily.

I have been taking Optivite and Evening Primrose for the menopause, but find that Optivite suits me best (I am 52 years old). Please tell me how many tablets I ought to be taking?
Take one tablet of Optivite three times a day.

I am in the menopause and would like to know how cervical polyps should be treated?
Try taking 15 drops of Petaforce twice daily after meals. If this does not have the required effect, contact a qualified practitioner, who may be able to advise you further after having been informed of your medical details.

I know that the menopause is not a disease, yet it is difficult to cope with. How can a woman help herself to prepare for and live through it?
You must always consider this phase of life in a positive light. Read the answers to some of the other questions in this section and also read my book *Menopause*.

Can calcium be taken during or after the menopause to prevent osteoporosis instead of HRT?
In many cases a calcium preparation is sufficient and I usually recommend that it is taken in combination with Oil of Evening Primrose. However, if osteoporosis is already present I would also suggest taking OstcoPrime from Enzymatic Therapy.

Which remedy do you recommend for heavy periods and acute period pains (during the early stages of the menopause)? I have tried Oil of Evening Primrose, but this does not ease the problem.
Twice a day, take 15 drops of Dr Vogel's MNP Formula together with one tablet of Sepia.

What can be done for thinning hair in menopausal women?
Take one tablet of Health Insurance Plus, together with five tablets of Urticalcin, both twice daily.

MIGRAINES

Could you please explain about migraine headaches, e.g. the causes and remedies?
This is a near enough impossible task because there are numerous types of migraines. Someone once tried to list them and reached 36 different types. The most common migraines are caused by allergies, cervical disalignments, gallbladder or liver problems or malfunctions, digestive disorders and hormonal problems. An accurate diagnosis must first be obtained before the correct treatment can be prescribed. I would suggest that for more detailed information you read my book *Migraine and Epilepsy*.

I suffer from migraines so often that I despair. What can I do?
I must repeat that the precise cause must be found in order to be able to prescribe the correct treatment. After a diagnosis has been reached you could consult either a specialist, an osteopath or an acupuncturist.

With respect to remedies, I would suggest you try Dr Vogel's Migraine Formula, and as an alternative for painkillers you could take either Petadolor or Petaforce.

I have very severe migraine attacks every 2–3 weeks, usually lasting for three days. I eat a healthy diet and do not drink coffee or alcohol; nor do I smoke. What can I do?
Take Dr Vogel's Migraine Formula twice daily and ban from your diet all cheese, wine, citrus fruits and chocolate.

More or less as long as I can remember I have experienced bad migraines. Before my child was born I attended the homoeopathic hospital and have tried everything. I have even been to faith healers, but all to no avail. Can you please help?
Once again, I must stress that the correct diagnosis must be obtained. If you have not found an answer in homoeopathy, try another form of alternative medicine, e.g. acupuncture or herbal remedies. It is, however, of the utmost importance to find the root of the problem.

My wife still gets bad migraines, even though she no longer menstruates. Can you explain this please?
It should be understood that migraines are not always related to the hormonal system. There can be a host of other reasons. Suggest to your wife that she visits a well-qualified practitioner, who may help to get to the root of the problem.

I would like to hear your opinion regarding acupuncture treatment for migraines. I am undergoing such a course at the moment and feel that it is being quite successful, although I agree it is still early days. I don't yet know if this will supply a permanent solution. Do you think that some time in the future this kind of treatment may become available on the NHS? I have also tried BUPA, but have had no joy there either.

I have been in practice a long time now and in that time I have seen some great recoveries by migraine patients, thanks to acupuncture. Therefore you should aim to finish your course.

With regard to the second part of your question, I firmly believe that the treatment should be made available by the NHS. Patients should demand it because many savings could be made. Occasionally I have encountered a BUPA patient who was allowed to claim the cost of the treatment, and the PPP medical policy has allowed the treatment to be refunded. It all depends on the type of policy you have.

What dietary measures would you suggest for migraine headaches?

In the initial stages of the treatment I would look for allergic reactions. In most cases migraine patients cannot tolerate chocolate, cheese, wine and citrus fruits. Try to eliminate these foodstuffs from the diet and also take 15 drops of Dr Vogel's Migraine Formula twice daily.

I frequently have a bad migraine – always down the side of the left eye. Can anything be done about this condition without the need to take drugs?

Try the homoeopathic remedies *Thuja 6x* or *Spigelia 6x*. If these are ineffective please seek the personal attention of an alternative practitioner, who may be able to do some tests.

Do you have a solution or some advice for migraine headaches that occur especially during menstruation?

It is important to know the exact timing of the migraine in relation to the menstrual cycle, as the advice for treating migraines that occur before the menstrual period may vary from that for migraines that strike after menstruation. However, in all cases Venosan will be beneficial and for more detailed advice I would suggest that you read my books *Menstrual and Pre-Menstrual Tension* and *Migraine and Epilepsy*. In either publication you will find some useful general advice.

How can a migraine sufferer help oneself?

Take plenty of fresh air and follow a wholesome diet. Follow your practitioner's advice and take the prescribed remedies faithfully. Finally, have you ever tried the natural remedy Feverfew?

I suffer with menstrual migraines. I have even had a hysterectomy and I still get them. They last for about 3–5 days. For three months I have been on a hormone treatment, which was a nasal spray containing Buserelin, but this made me worse. I wonder if you can recommend any treatment that can help me?

Take PMS Formula one week before your period is due. Then take ten drops of *Loranthus* twice daily.

I would like to know if it is common for a child to suffer constantly with abdominal migraine? My granddaughter is twelve years old and has been suffering with this since she was six. For the last year she has been under constant treatment.

I must say that this condition is not common among children of that age and she certainly needs help. Please read my book *Migraine and Epilepsy* for some general advice for such cases.

MOTOR NEURONE DISEASE

What is motor neurone disease?

This is a progressive degeneration of the nerves that deliver messages to the muscles of the body. The symptoms of this disease are muscle degeneration, weakness and wasting, often accompanied by difficulty in walking, swallowing and breathing.

My mother has been diagnosed as having motor neurone disease. Do you believe that this condition is caused by an imbalance in the endocrine system and do you believe that the degenerative process can be either halted or reversed?

Considering some recent successes with the use of amino acids for patients with motor neurone disease, it definitely would seem that the endocrine system is involved. Much research is taking place in the cause and treatment of this disease and much still remains to be learned.

My niece's husband (aged 33) was diagnosed as having motor neurone disease two months ago. The family is looking everywhere for help, knowing that, as yet, there is no cure.

What homoeopathic treatment could he try?
There are some homoeopathic remedies that might help, but they need to be prescribed by a practitioner who has had the opportunity to examine the patient first. Such a practitioner will also advise on dietary guidelines. Electro-acupuncture is often beneficial.

MULTIPLE SCLEROSIS (MS)

A friend of mine is undergoing tests to ascertain whether she suffers from multiple sclerosis. Can you tell me some more about this illness?
Multiple sclerosis (MS) is a condition where nerve fibres in the central nervous system become damaged, caused by inflammation of the fatty tissue (myelin) which insulates and covers them. In some cases it can be a crippling disease, while other patients experience double vision, numbness, difficulty with urinating, imbalance when walking and unsteadiness of the legs. More detailed information can be found in my book *Multiple Sclerosis*.

Do orthodox medications, e.g. Prednisilone or cortisone, enhance the chances of recovery for MS patients?
Cortisone and Prednisilone are often prescribed for multiple sclerosis. Sometimes they are needed – sometimes they are helpful – but I much prefer alternative treatment methods because they are less harsh and the risk of side-effects is cancelled.

The programme I use for my patients has been worked out with Roger McDougall and is as follows:

1. A gluten-free diet.
2. Use of supplementary vitamins, minerals and trace elements.
3. Hydrotherapy.
4. Acupuncture treatment.

What can be done for multiple sclerosis?
First of all it should be understood that one should not give in to this condition, but keep fighting it. For detailed advice on how this can be done please read my book *Multiple Sclerosis*.

I have a friend who has had MS for 12 years now. What herbs will be of help to her?
There are several herbs that are of benefit to MS patients, dependent upon the specific condition and the symptoms experienced. The main symptoms are circulation problems, for which I prescribe *Hypericum*, and for bladder weakness your friend should try *Solidago* or a complex herbal remedy called Cystoforce.

What kind of treatments are recommended for MS patients?
Please read the answer to an earlier question where I listed the four main components of my programme for multiple sclerosis patients. Sometimes osteopathy, reflexology or aromatherapy can also be included in this programme.

Does stress exacerbate multiple sclerosis symptoms?
There is no doubt that stress will generally have an adverse impact on Multiple Sclerosis sufferers.

Do you know any method for relieving the pain caused by multiple sclerosis?
It is rare for MS patients to complain about pain. If they do, it is usually because of circulatory problems, and in such cases I mostly prescribe *Hypericum*.

Which preparations would you recommend for a 40-year-old male with MS?
Many of my patients have reported a considerable improvement in their condition as a result of treatment with a full spectrum of amino acids. Please see a qualified practitioner for more details of this treatment method.

Can anything be done to overcome a gluten intolerance?
This is very unlikely. However, Professor Roger McDougall has put together a very good gluten-free diet and comprehensive details of this can be found in my book *Multiple Sclerosis*.

I have multiple sclerosis and have read your book on the subject. I have adopted the Roger McDougall diet and have made progress. I want to know if I can achieve any further

improvement and would ask you if I should book regular sessions with yourself?

Besides following the Roger McDougall dietary guidelines, the four main points of the programme also include supplementary vitamins and minerals, hydrotherapy and, where possible, acupuncture treatment. On that basis I would be more than happy to advise you on a personal basis.

My friend suffers from MS. She also has a heart condition. Then recently she developed a rare skin disease called erythema multi-form. She has been put on steroids four times to ease the pain, but the doctors do not seem to treat the problem. Could you please advise her?

This condition, which manifests itself as an acute eruption of the skin, may follow tonsilitis, or may be associated with acute rheumatism, tuberculosis (*Herpes*) cold sores or a blood syndrome, and many cases come into the category of a virus of unknown origin. It can be treated homoeopathically and therefore your friend should find an experienced homoeopathic practitioner who may be able to diagnose the viral condition with the use of a Vega-Mora or Vincent machine.

What can a person do in the early stages of MS to prevent further deterioration? I have had a benign condition for 15 years, but am now having an acceleration.

No one can ever tell how long a remission will last. Some people's condition never progresses to the more serious phases of multiple sclerosis, while others never seem to enjoy a period of remission. My advice to your question as to how further deterioration may be prevented is to follow Professor Roger McDougall's dietary guidelines and also use supplementary vitamin mineral and trace element preparations. You can find more advice in my book *Multiple Sclerosis*.

I have MS. Would electro-acupuncture help to overcome double vision and poor balance?

Many people with your symptoms have greatly benefited from electro-acupuncture with light colour therapy. Please consult a qualified practitioner for more individual advice.

What can you tell me about hereditary factors in illnesses such as MS, muscular dystrophy, diabetes, etc?

This is a very difficult question, because only by tracing a family's medical history can it be answered. It seems that by tracing the medical history of a muscular dystrophy patient a hereditary link is sometimes found.

I would like you to know that when I was 32 I had multiple sclerosis and was given one year to live. I have had homoeopathic treatment for 12 years, dealing with paralysis and blindness in one eye. My sight returned after 18 months and as the treatment progressed the remissions became longer. Since the age of 45 I have had no sign of this disease and I will be 72 next birthday. The only thing left is a 'low pain threshold', e.g. it hurts when I fall off my bicycle!
Your experience is proof of the power of positive thinking. Well done – and may you long continue to enjoy the good health you deserve!

Could I have some advice for a person in my exercise class who suffers from multiple sclerosis? I would like to know what type of exercises to avoid and what would benefit her most.
Strenuous exercises should be avoided. Teach her some gentle stretching exercises and recommend cycling, swimming and walking.

Would an MS patient benefit from a straight oxygen intake each day? At present she is doing deep-breathing exercises.
No, the intake of straight oxygen is not advisable. If an oxygen treatment has been decided upon, this may only be undertaken under medical supervision. Please seek specialist advice, because safe oxygen treatment methods do exist; in particular, some very good results have been achieved with hyperbaric oxygen treatment.

What, if anything, is new in the treatment of multiple sclerosis?
The latest development is Beta-Interferon, but research is still taking place. At the moment this treatment is not widely available on the NHS or from alternative practitioners. It is also very expensive.

MUSCLE PAIN

I have so much muscle pain every day. What can I do?
Rub the affected areas with either Toxeucal Oil or Symphytum officinalis.

MYALGIC ENCEPHALOMYELITIS (ME)

Exactly what does the term ME mean?
ME is the abbreviation for myalgic encephalomyelitis – also known as
'post-viral syndrome' or 'Yuppie Flu' – which condition describes a viral
attack on the immune system. Many ME patients have previously suffered
from an attack of glandular fever that has not been correctly treated.
During recuperation any viral attacks should be taken seriously and
according to the homoeopathic principles any illness should go through a
'healing crisis' in order to enable the system to overcome the illness, its
side-effects or influences. Myalgic encephalomyelitis is variously
symptomised by extreme tiredness, headaches, abdominal pains, cold
extremities, panic attacks, numbness, muscle pains and depression.

**I would much appreciate any advice on 'post-viral
syndrome'. Typical symptoms in my case are lethargy/
tiredness, memory loss, muscle pains, frequent throat
infections and depression. At present I attend a homoeopathic hospital, where I have been advised to take Co-enzyme
Q10, Evening Primrose Oil, multivitamins and ginseng.**
You already have taken some very sensible steps by following the advice
given by your homoeopathic practitioner. Depending upon the situation,
I sometimes also recommend *Ginkgo biloba* and Imuno-Strength. Finally
always remain positive and continue to believe that you will overcome this
condition.

**What advice would you give to a female ME sufferer in her
mid-forties? At the age of 36 I was diagnosed with breast
cancer, which was treated in the traditional fashion, i.e. 'cut-
burn-poison'. I very much prefer alternative treatment
methods.**
With your medical history you would be well advised to seek specialist

guidance. Please read my books *Cancer and Leukaemia*, and *Viruses, Allergies and the Immune System*, where you will find much useful advice.

I would very much like to know if you can recommend any forms of treatment for the symptoms of ME?

It should be understood that even though some of the symptoms are present in most ME sufferers, the treatment may vary greatly from one patient to another. Some patients benefit from acupuncture, others from homoeopathy, herbal treatment or metabolic therapy. Soft-tissue massage helps some patients; others benefit from reflexology or aromatherapy. As you can see, different approaches work for different patients. One thing that all ME patients have in common is that they all benefit from sympathy and understanding.

What advice would you give to people with ME symptoms and how do you feel about amalgam dental fillings? I would also be curious to learn your opinion on the Bach Flower remedies.

General advice on how to deal with ME symptoms has already been given in the answer to the previous questions. With relation to amalgam dental fillings, I would say that I very much prefer porcelain or composite fillings and quite a number of my patients have shown considerable improvement after having their amalgam fillings removed. As for the last part of your question, treatment with Bach Flower remedies is usually considered in a very favourable light, by myself included.

My daughter has had ME for over a year. The doctor at the hospital has recommended Efamol (containing Evening Primrose and fish extracts). Does she need to take codliver oil with this and should she show improvement in one month?

In some cases it is indeed preferable to use a combination remedy of evening primrose oil and fish oil, but you or your daughter will be disappointed if you seriously expect to see some results within the span of one month. ME is a very persistent condition and it will take considerably longer before any lasting improvement will be noticeable.

Can you advise on remedies for ME (or 'Yuppie Flu')?

The term 'Yuppie flu' originates from the USA, probably as it used to be very much associated with glandular fever. It is interesting to note that yet another term used in the United States for ME is 'the kissing disease'. The use of these terms in relation to ME has mostly disappeared now, as the disease has unfortunately grown more common and is more widely recognised. I would suggest that you read my book *Viruses, Allergies and the Immune System* for general advice.

What are your thoughts on a link between hyperventilation and ME? If there is a link, which comes first? My skin is tinged with yellow and this is said to be caused by ME, but nothing abnormal has been found in my blood. Since I was diagnosed as having ME my blood pressure has been low: 90 over low 50s. Please inform me regarding some possible causes and remedies.

Some ME patients do have problems with hyperventilation, but usually the ME condition comes first, with hyperventilation being a possible symptom. Usually, the colour of the skin depends on how tired the patient is. Make sure that your diet contains plenty of fresh foods, including plenty of fruit and vegetables. As you have not given an indication of your age, I cannot comment on your blood pressure. However, if it has risen or dropped from its normal level, there are remedies that can be taken to balance this.

Six years ago I had a virus and immediately afterwards I developed a considerable number of food allergies. Although my general health has improved since then, the number of foods which upset me has increased. I am on a rotary-diversified diet which excludes the worst offenders. Are you able to suggest a way of improving the situation? I do eat a very good nutritious diet.

Some foods cause irritable bowel syndrome and others cause headaches, fatigue and sore or stiff joints and muscles, or possibly ME.

When the immune system is attacked allergies often become apparent and one can become allergic to almost anything. Take all possible measures to strengthen your immune system. For this purpose I would suggest that you read my book *Viruses, Allergies and the Immune System* as well as reading the section on the immune system in this book (pages 127-9).

Can the group of ME viruses be eventually passed out through the system or do they stay within the body and become inactive?

The body is a wonderful natural invention and is comparable to a complicated biochemical laboratory. Thank goodness that this effective system is often able to rid itself of invading enemies.

Which consumption product causes ME?

It is very difficult to tell what exactly causes ME, but the general belief is that it is virus-induced. Despite this, I would still suggest that diet is taken into account and my recommendation would be to ensure that the diet consists of mainly fresh foods, including plenty of vegetables and fruit.

On the subject of ME, could you tell me if any permanent or irreversible damage is caused by this disease, e.g. damage to the central nervous system?

Thankfully, I have only come across one or two cases where I have been in doubt as to the long-term or permanent effect of any damage inflicted. These were very severe cases of ME and yet, even then I could not rule out the possibility that the damage could be overcome.

What remedy do you recommend for ME sufferers to relieve painful symptoms? When deep depression exists, would you support the use of anti–depressant drugs? What herbal remedies could be used to boost the immune system and increase hormone secretion?

To boost the immune system I would prescribe three Imuno-Strength tablets daily, and 15 drops of the herbal remedy *Ginkgo biloba* twice daily. To balance the hormonal system take three 500 mg capsules of Oil of Evening Primrose daily.

What is the main thing that I can do to help my husband, who has ME? Fortunately, he is improving greatly at present and this improvement set in when I started doing reflexology on him. However, he still gets periods of intense fatigue.

As he is already improving I would continue with the treatment therapies he uses at present. Perhaps you can give him some extra help with Imuno-Strength and *Ginkgo biloba*.

How much vitamin C should ME patients take?

As a rule, ME patients should take 2–4 g of vitamin C daily.

My son has had ME for four years now. After the first three years he turned to alternative treatment. He has been on a wheat-free rotation diet, for the last six months, and now his diet is also sugar-free and yeast-free. Over the last year he has taken much medication, i.e. Health Insurance Plus, pantothenic acid, vitamin C, magnesium and Mycocidin – all on a daily basis in varying strengths. As yet there is no improvement. He has been at home since he became ill; he is unable to study or work as he is always so tired. I am rather concerned about all this medication. Could it be harmful if taken over a long period? How long should he continue with the treatment if there is no improvement?

Please do not worry unnecessarily, because he is not taking too much medication. However, I would have expected there to have been some improvement and a general suggestion would be that he also take *Ginkgo biloba* and Thymuplex. Furthermore, I would suggest that he place himself under the guidance of a fully qualified practitioner, who can advise him on a personal basis.

I have heard that antibiotics have an adverse effect on ME. Why is this?

Antibiotics often cause side-effects and this is primarily because the good bacteria are destroyed along with the bad bacteria.

How many Oil of Evening Primrose capsules should an ME patient take daily?

In general the recommendation is three 500 mg capsules daily, to be taken half an hour to one hour before going to bed.

Could ME be caused by family problems and emotional stress?

Stress and emotional upsets always lower one's resistance and affect the immune system. This allows a person to become more susceptible to invading bacteria or viruses.

What are the usual symptoms of ME?

Typical symptoms of ME include tiredness, feeling bloated, muscle pains, shoulder tension, cold and hot sweats, nervousness and depression.

What is your opinion of Dr Behan's research and treatment of ME?

From the case histories I have read, I am very impressed with his work in this field.

In your experience has there ever been a time in the treatment of an ME patient that you have been able to say: 'You are cured!'?

The capacity to cure lies within oneself, but I am pleased to say that among my patients I have many completely recovered ME sufferers.

Could you comment on a possible relationship between ME and 'zapping' (electronic pollution)?

Unfortunately, any kind of pollution is detrimental to ME patients and the general rule must be to keep food and environment as natural as possible.

What advice do you have for the ME sufferer regarding exercise? Could it be possible for example, that the ME sufferer fails to improve because he or she is not strengthening the muscles sufficiently? Conversely, can over-exercise have a damaging effect?

Exercise such as swimming, walking or cycling is very good, but do not over-exercise. The exercise methods mentioned need not be strenuous, and when you become tired there is no harm at all in taking a rest. Remember that fresh air is essential.

Last year I had pains in the chest and stomach. Tests concluded that they were due to a virus which was there 'to stay' and the pains occasionally recur. The only treatment suggested is steroids, which I do not want. I am permanently tired, yet sleep like a log. Is there any appropriate homoeopathic treatment?

It sounds as if you may have ME but I would hasten to add that it is time you had your complaints properly diagnosed. Until then it is just guesswork and therefore impossible for any practitioner to prescribe appropriate remedies or treatment methods.

Could you please elaborate on the term 'healing crisis'?
All illness and disease has to pass through a crisis. Naturopathy and homoeopathy try to remove the cause of the illness or disease from the system, and this often results in a period of fever, with a rise in temperature and sweats. This is often referred to as the 'healing crisis'.

Is there a vitamin supplement to help ME? I have severe muscle spasms and these sometimes wake me in the night. For me the most distressing symptom is the brain fatigue and my poor memory. I have a feeling of pressure at the back of my head and neck and also experience muscle pain and exhaustion. My other symptoms include sweating at night and a low body temperature. I have changed my diet to include many whole foods and would like to know what else I should do.
Please take Imuno-Strength every day and for the muscle pain take two capsules of Seatone twice a day. For general advice read my book *Viruses, Allergies and the Immune System*.

For the last 2–3 years I have been very ill with ME. My doctor believes it began with a virus called Bonn Holmes' disease. However, I have wondered if it is hormone-related, as I feel I have never been right since the birth of my second child 11 years ago. Since then I have suffered from severe pre-menstrual tension and feel that I have gradually deteriorated.
Certain tests have shown a variable hormonal output. In the case of Interleukin one can definitely subscribe to hormonal imbalance in ME patients and this link is at present being investigated.

Now that ME is more widely recognised, what do you think is the main contributing factor according to your own observations while treating people long-term?
The main factor in a case of ME, to my mind, is the lowering of the immune system as a result of previous viral or bacterial infections or influences. The World Health Organisation has categorised ME as a disease of the nervous system, but I feel strongly that it is interrelated to the immune system.

What is the latest recommended treatment for chronic fatigue?

In our clinic we have recently begun to use a substance called Coneflower Extract together with Coliacron injections, and the initial feedback is very encouraging.

On the subject of chronic fatigue syndrome, what do you think would relieve muscle aching or fibromyalgia?

It is not unusual for ME patients to have fibromyalgia complaints. I have obtained the best results with homoeopuncture, which is a combination treatment of acupuncture and homoeopathy.

Do you think that if the body's own electromagnetic forces are out of balance, or indeed are subject to interference by outside electromagnetic or other atmospheric changes, that this in turn can cause problems with the immune system, e.g. ME? I have had ME for six years and over the past two years another three people I know of, who also have ME, have had relapses at the same time as me. These are people I do not frequently see. I have always felt that external factors of this type can influence the body's own 'energy' and are perhaps instrumental in many conditions (mental and physical). P.S. The treatment I receive at your clinic enables me to lead a fairly normal life.

Although the assumptions in your question have not been proven, I have seen a number of people with geopathic stress indications. Sometimes I can group ME patients into geographical patterns, which leads me to wonder what influences are involved. I do not doubt that electromagnetic influences can affect the immune system.

Why would the left side of the body be more painful and sore in a person suffering from ME?

This is dependent upon the flow of the energy in the body of the individual. Each person is different and will be affected in a slightly different manner. The 'yin' and 'yang' life streams should be in balance – in other words the negative and positive energy channels. In your case it sounds as if there is a blockage on the left side. Consult a qualified acupuncturist, who will be able to clear the blockage and help to restore the immune system.

How do you dissolve amalgam? A friend of mine was a dental

assistant and she rolled the amalgam in her bare hands. She is still fighting to regain her health. Can amalgam cause ME?

Dental amalgam is a blend of the alloy mercury with silver, and has only recently been recognised as a possible, or even likely, detrimental influence on general health. If in doubt I will always advise patients to gradually have these fillings removed and replaced with composite fillings. I have seen very marked improvements in the condition of some of my patients after the amalgam fillings had been removed.

I have heard that the ME virus can be genetically imprinted. Is this true? If this were the case, can the ME virus play a part in pregnancy and become a hereditary factor?

It must be understood that all human beings carry the seeds of degeneration from birth. The most important thing is to realise that by looking after our immune system we can effect certain changes, and therefore I always stress that any infection, viral attack or inflamed condition should be treated. Having said all this, I must add that I have never heard of the ME virus being passed on to a baby prior to its birth.

I would like to know what your views are on the chronic fatigue in ME sufferers? I have had ME for five years and am still unable to return to work.

In cases of ME it can be a very long time before a change in the condition is noticeable. Yet I have seen patients who reported many years of no change or even a change for the worse subsequently make a full recovery. It is essential to keep a positive frame of mind at all times, even though this may not always be easy. Please read my book *Viruses, Allergies and the Immune System* for further advice.

My daughter has been suffering from ME for some time now and I wonder if you could advise what she can take to relieve the pain?

Fortunately, few ME patients complain about pain associated with this disease. The most common complaint is the excessive tiredness and lethargy they experience. However, if the pain is associated with ME, I would suggest that your daughter take two tablets of Petaforce twice daily.

What do you feel about ingesting hydrogen peroxide for chronic fatigue syndrome?

Hydrogen peroxide treatment requires the strict supervision of a qualified practitioner and should only be undertaken with extreme care. I would much prefer to see it used in the form of a weak solution, as a throat gargle.

My husband has had a virus for several months which causes the glands in his neck and chin to swell. When these glands become prominent or noticeable he always feels exhausted. Could this possibly be ME? Can you advise on what to do?
There are many people who would suspect the same diagnosis under these circumstances, but for ME to be properly diagnosed it needs further investigation. Until an actual diagnosis has been reached it is very difficult to advise on a treatment method.

I am an ME patient and I would like to know if you could advise specifically on ways to improve my sleeping cycle? I cannot sleep and feel worse as a result and then the tiredness gets me down. It feels like I am going round in circles.
I sympathise with you because irregular sleep is in itself very tiresome. Try taking three capsules of Oil of Evening Primrose before going to bed. Alternatively, you could take 30 drops of Dormeasan one hour before retiring.

My son has a low-level viral infection (ME syndrome). He has had this for three years and is receiving medication from the doctor, but we wonder if you could help?
Unfortunately, it is often the case that this disease affects young people and changes their life. All too frequently I hear of youngsters not being able to complete their studies because of ME and all this will have a lasting effect in later years. Please read my book *Viruses, Allergies and the Immune System*, and with respect to specific remedies for young people, I often prescribe the following programme: CPS Formula (an enzyme product), *Ginkgo biloba* (a herbal remedy) and Imuno-Strength (a vitamin, mineral and trace element supplement).

Is there anything you can suggest to help my 17-year-old son, who is suffering from ME? He has been taking multivitamins and minerals, which are a great help, but still finds it too exhausting to cope with things. He tried to go back to his studies without success.

Thank goodness, at least you have started him off with supplementary vitamins and minerals, but he will need more than that. As ME patients often appear to have active *Candida* problems too, a good cleansing programme is usually beneficial, as is a fresh look at the diet. Depending upon the severity of the disease, magnesium or enzyme injections may be required.

To help the body to rid itself of viruses or miasmas, *Harpagophytum* should be taken, sometimes combined with Oil of Evening Primrose and/or *Ginkgo biloba*.

N

NAIL PROBLEMS

What would you advise for fungus under the nails?
Try to carefully dab on some *Spilanthes* between the nails and the skin of the fingers or toes. Using a little cottonwool wrapped around a cocktail stick may be the best way to do this.

What causes nail ridges? Is there a remedy?
Rub the nails with warm olive oil and take five tablets of Urticalcin twice daily.

My nails have ridges and they crack, chip and refuse to grow. What does this indicate and what should I do about it?
This is probably due to a deficiency of silicia and calcium, and these minerals can be replenished by taking a supplement.

What causes vertical lines on one's nails?
I would suggest that you consult a practitioner to check out this symptom, because without further information I cannot advise you safely.

What does it mean when the nails are dumpy like waves and what do ridges mean?
Take five tablets of Urticalcin twice daily to overcome a probable calcium deficiency and also regularly rub the nails together.

NERVOUS COMPLAINTS AND DISORDERS

Lately I have been feeling nervous and irritated every day and I do not know what causes it.

Life should be enjoyed and that is impossible if you feel tense and nervous, especially if you do not know the reason for feeling as you do. Take 15 drops of *Avena sativa* and one tablet of Ginsavita twice daily. If there is no improvement you should discuss your symptoms with a doctor or practitioner.

If somebody has an emotional problem, and cannot get along with other, annoying, people and as a result is rejected in a group situation, people do not want that person's company. What would you suggest for him or her?
Firstly, I would advise that the person reads my book *Stress and Nervous Disorders*, because I often hear how much the advice it contains has helped people with similar complaints. To overcome emotional problems some suitable homoeopathic remedies are zinc, Valerian, *Tanatia* or *Avena sativa*.

I feel so unsettled no matter where I go. I feel as if I have been uprooted all my life. I am trying very hard to settle down in a new house and new town, but so many things get on my nerves and my confidence goes. I can't sleep properly and have upsetting dreams. I wake up with headaches and sore and hot eyes, feeling very tired. I have palpitations and my neck and shoulders ache. Some days I feel OK and I can cope, but other days I just don't know what is wrong with me. I am beginning to think that I am mentally unbalanced.
Please, no more talk like that – I don't think that you are mentally unbalanced. You just need some help and you should have asked for help sooner, before you reached this deep depression and lack of confidence.

Firstly, I would prescribe a constitutional remedy, *Argentum nitricum*, for three days, to be followed for two days by Aconite. Then, on a longer-term basis, take two tablets of Ginsavita together with two tablets of Neuroforce twice daily. I am convinced that you will soon see a change for the better.

What can you suggest as treatment for a depression following the death of my husband and moving house? Can you help me overcome feelings of insecurity?
For a month take 15 drops of *Ignatia D3* twice daily. Thereafter, take 15 drops of Hyperiforce, also twice daily.

My husband is retired and in his mid sixties. He has suffered all his life with shouting or getting violent in his sleep (sometimes he even falls out of bed), usually at about 5.30 in the morning, which disturbs the rest of the family. He is a good sleeper and it does not disturb him. He is against taking any form of drugs, even sleeping tablets. He leads a normal, quiet, life. Is there a suitable herbal remedy?

There is a marvellous herb called Kava Kava, which he should take, and before going to bed give him 30 drops of Dormeasan.

Is there any one homoeopathic remedy for stress on a long-term basis, i.e. nerves?

Take 15 drops of *Avena sativa* twice daily, together with two Jayvee tablets, also twice daily. Although I believe that an adequate diet and sufficient rest are essential for good health, I recognise that life is very demanding for a large proportion of the population, who may need natural extra help. Jayvee is a formulation that can be used without fear of unpleasant side-effects or addiction. It contains a blend of substances known to have soothing properties, including *Valeriana, Crataegus* (hawthorn), *Humulus lupulus* (hop), *Viscum album* (mistletoe), *Passiflora*, *Melissa* (lemon balm) and zinc (which combines well with valerian).

Can you recommend any herbs or herbal preparations for stress?

Suitable herbs to ease the symptoms of stress include *Avena sativa*, ginseng, *Valeriana, Melissa* and hops.

Can you suggest anything to help a person who suffers with mood swings?

Mood swings can be caused by many influences or reasons and rather than just taking a remedy, you should try to get to the cause of it. A remedy called RelaxoZyme from Enzymatic Therapy has helped many people, but I must emphasise that you should try and find the underlying reason for your mood swings.

What can a person do for anxiety and panic attacks?

First of all I would suggest that you read my book *Stress and Nervous Disorders* and practise the Hara breathing exercises which are described there. Also, take *Arnica 30x* for six days, to be followed by *Gelsemium 3x*.

When I do anything strenuous I feel faint, go dry in the mouth and my eye sight is affected. When I am in bed I ache all over, especially in the groin, where I feel strong pressure on the right testicle. I pass water three or four times a night and if I suppress the urge I get pains. I become very tired and stressed over nothing.

Seek osteopathic treatment and practise some relaxation exercises. Also, take two tablets of Ginsavita twice daily.

What would you suggest for nervous tremors, muscle spasms and cramp? Would you advise CoQ10 enzyme?

CoQ10 is an excellent remedy to use in such cases. However, I also feel that you would benefit from acupuncture.

What do you suggest for feelings of tiredness, depression, emotional anxiety and loss of joie de vivre? I am 44 years of age.

You need a good 'pick-me-up'. Twice daily, take 15 drops of Hyperiforce, together with Vitaforce and Escalation Formula from Enzymatic Therapy.

I would like anyone who has been on tranquillisers long-term to know that it is possible to come off them. I was on them for 15 years and it took me a whole year to get off them, but life is a lot better now.

Positive action from this lady greatly improved her life. Remember that there are many alternative remedies to help people to overcome such an addiction, without any lasting side-effects.

Fourteen years ago three close relatives died and I was put on tranquillisers. I have been told that I am hooked and cannot give them up. Can you help?

Of course it is possible to overcome this habit. Surely you do not want to be dependent on these pills for the rest of your life? You must not, however, throw the pills out and try to do it overnight. It would make more sense to consult a practitioner and use some herbal substitutes, e.g. *Avena sativa*, Hyperiforce and *Passiflora*.

My son is 27 years old and suffers from palpitations and over-breathing. He cannot always catch his breath. Can you recommend anything to help him?

The problems you describe are sometimes linked with hyperventilation. Give your son Aconite 30x every day for about one week, and see if the symptoms disappear. If they do not, seek the help of an alternative practitioner.

Can homoeopathic medicine help to overcome phobias and fears?

Yes, it certainly can. I cannot make any recommendation without knowing more details, but I would suggest that you find yourself a qualified practitioner and explain your problems.

What foods should I avoid if I suffer from anxiety which is not self-induced but occurs regularly, varying in severity, but sometimes lasting for three weeks?

Follow the low-stress diet prescribed in my book *Stress and Nervous Disorders.*

Could you please advise on tension symptoms, particularly aches at the back of the head?

If there is any tension at all, it will nearly always display itself in the head in some ache or pain. The head carries more tension than any other part of the body. In such cases osteopathic treatment will often be most helpful.

My sister had been on tranquillisers for ten years and four months ago she, thankfully, managed to come off them. She is now very weak and wonders if you can recommend any remedies?

Tell your sister to take two tablespoons of Vitaforce and two tablets of Imuno-Strength daily.

My mother will be 70 next week and she is overweight, cynical, depressed, never really well and suffers from arthritis and diverticulitis, also a chronic urine infection. What can I give her that might help her, despite herself?

Give her two Jayvee tablets twice daily. For the depression she needs 15 drops of *Hypericum perforatum* twice daily and for the arthritis 15 drops of Imperthritica twice daily. Good luck!

I am a nervous person and would like to know if fear of flying can be overcome?
Yes, I have seen marvellous results with the Rescue Remedy from Dr Bach. I would also suggest that you try some acupuncture treatment.

Is an aversion to loud noises – even loud conversation, for example in a restaurant – a sign of anything specific?
You may feel stressed and therefore have less tolerance to noise. Take Aconite 3x for three days, and then take Zinc 3x.

What do you recommend for depression (caused by a brain chemical imbalance)?
Read my book *Stress and Nervous Disorders* for general advice and also take supplementary zinc, Valerian and Jayvee tablets.

NEURALGIA

Is there a remedy for neuralgia?
The very best results for neuralgia I have seen when using the homoeopathic remedy *Marum verum* (15 drops twice daily).

I have had trigeminal neuralgia for two years and I am experiencing very severe headaches and sore and tired eyes. Is it my condition that is affecting my eyes?
Indeed, it is very likely that your eye complaints are caused by your condition. Start using Petaforce as soon as possible (ten drops twice daily). Acupuncture or laser treatment can also be highly beneficial in such cases.

NUTRITION

In your opinion, what is the best food?
The only way I can answer that question is that the best type of food must be those foods that were originally given to mankind for eating: fruits, vegetables and nuts. These should always be the main components of our daily food intake. There are many other kinds of food that man has introduced over the centuries, which have left their marks on people's health.

Could you give a list of healing properties in foods?

Whenever possible, we should always look to our food for our nutritional needs. Never rely entirely on vitamin and mineral supplements, although these may be used to supplement our diet, especially when certain foods like vegetables or fruit are hard to obtain.

The following foods have been known to provide the nourishment needed for specific areas of the body or for treating specific ailments:

Apples	— for gallbladder and liver disorders, diarrhoea, constipation, loss of appetite
Apricots	— detoxify the liver and pancreas
Asparagus	— for fatty tumours and urinary secretions
Avocado	— a fat and protein supplier; good for diabetics
Barley	— a calcium supplier; aids the colon; a lymph cleanser
Beans (green)	— remove metallic poison; good for the pancreas
Beans (Lima)	— combat drugs residues
Blueberries	— feed the pancreas; for sugar problems
Beef	— a muscle food
Beets	— a spleen food
Cabbage	— supplies vitamin C, the tissue builder
Carrots	— for the eyes, blood and lymph
Chicken	— a gland food
Cucumber	— a skin remedy, kidney cleanser and infection cleanser
Figs	— a de-wormer
Fish	— a good protein and iodine supplier
Garlic	— for carbohydrates residue in tissue and glands
Grapefruit	— a lime supplier; for flu
Lemon	— supplies vitamin C; strengthens tissue
Lentils	— supply iron and protein
Millet	— the 'meat' of vegetarians (15 per cent protein)
Oats	— a brain food
Oils (cold-pressed)	— required to assimilate the proteins from vegetables; a kidney food
Okra	— regulates female bleeding; gives strength to leukaemia sufferers
Onion	— for flu

Oranges	— vitamin C; flu prevention
Papaya	— for protein digestion
Peas	— supplies protein; good for weak stomachs
Pineapple	— an enzyme supplier
Pomegranate	— a de-wormer
Potatoes (red)	— for stomach and duodenal ulcers
Prunes	— supply iron; for constipation
Pumpkin	— a de-wormer; a spleen and pancreas food
Radishes	— promote the flow of bile
Raisins	— for anaemia; a blood builder
Rhubarb	— a colon cleanser
Rice gruel	— for diarrhoea
Sesame seeds	— an amino acid supplier
Spinach	— for anaemia
Sunflower seeds	— feed the eyes, sinuses, glands
Tomatoes	— for the liver; supply vitamin C
Turnips	— for deep-rooted tumours
Watermelon	— for sluggish kidneys and cleansing the kidneys
Yams	— a hormone food
Yoghurt	— for the necessary 'friendly' bacteria in the colon

What are nutritional deficiencies?

1. Do you have habitually stale or foul-smelling breath? This may indicate poor bowel function and insufficient fibre in the diet. Because we eat several times a day, if the food is being digested properly after each meal it should be starting to move through our system. We don't store our food for the day and eat it all at once, so eliminating waste only once a day could indicate that the food is moving through our system too slowly.

2. Does your hair seem to lack lustre? This may be due to deficiencies of biotin, amino acids or zinc. Amino acids are found in good-quality protein foods. If your diet lacks seeds, nuts, soya products, eggs or organic meats and poultry, it may also lack the correct balance of amino acids that are needed to rebuild cells and tissues. Healthy hair reflects health within the body.

3. Are your gums red or infected? Irritated gums may be the result of harsh chemicals in your toothpaste. Homoeopathic toothpastes are best

and are well tolerated by even the most sensitive people. Red or bleeding gums may indicate that vitamin C, zinc and folic acid levels are inadequate.

4. Is the skin at the back of your arms like sandpaper? A deficiency of vitamin A may cause this reaction. If you feel your intake is adequate, perhaps there is a malabsorption problem. Certain substances, especially caffeine found in coffee, cola, cocoa, chocolate or regular tea, may be destroying the digestive enzymes in your stomach so that the food cannot be broken down efficiently, the blood cannot be enriched and healing cannot take place. Dry skin cannot be corrected by creams and lotions alone, it must be nourished from within.

5. Do you feel weak, shaky or disorientated if you do not eat on time? This may indicate a blood sugar imbalance and possibly hypoglycaemia (low blood sugar). This does not mean that more sugar should be eaten in order to raise the sugar level; in fact, quite the opposite is true. Sugar should be completely eliminated from the diet and several smaller meals should be eaten throughout the day, rather than three large meals. A larger quantity of complex carbohydrates should be included in the diet.

6. Are you experiencing recurring constipation and/or diarrhoea? Check the fibre content in your diet. Fibre is not a laxative, but a regulator. If there is not enough, you may experience constipation – there is not enough bulk to move the waste matter through quickly enough. If you experience diarrhoea, extra fibre is also needed to soak up the excess moisture. Fruits and vegetables should be plentiful in the diet, along with whole grains.

7. Do you feel that stress is an overwhelming factor in your life? When the body is functioning properly, we feel we have all kinds of excess energy to help us cope with the stress we face. When even only a few areas in the body are out of balance, all our excess energy is directed towards keeping these organs working correctly and we begin to feel tired and unable to cope with any external stress. To the outside world, it may appear that the stress is causing the problem, but we know that when we begin to look within for imbalances and treat them, extra energy returns and stress no longer overwhelms us as it did before.

Could you give me some advice on children's dietary requirements please. My son won't eat meat at all, but eats fish and chicken. Does he need any mineral or vitamin supplements because of this?

In fact, your son is better off without meat, because meat is the hardest food to digest. However, make sure that he eats plenty of fresh fruit, vegetables, nuts and rice.

I have a four-year-old daughter who was never sick until the age of two. She now constantly has colds, swollen tonsils, fluid in her ears and a blocked nose. What can I do? (I take great care with her nutrition.)

Although you are conscious about nutrition, take a good look at her dairy food intake. Your daughter may have an allergy or she may have a deficiency of vitamins, minerals and trace elements. It also sounds as if she could do with an anti-congestion remedy and I would recommend that you give her a course of Echinaforce.

What is the best dietary regime for a child with learning difficulties?

Alway give children plenty of fruit and vegetables to eat. Also, from time to time give the child a few almonds to nibble. A suitable homoeopathic remedy is *Cerebrum*, which has often proved helpful under similar circumstances.

Are there any contra-indications to giving diet drinks to young children – in fairly large amounts?

Too much of anything is never a good thing. It depends what kinds of drinks you are referring to and also what you consider to be a 'fairly large amount'. Fruit juices cannot be harmful, but if the drinks you are referring to contain many additives and preservatives I would have to say that this cannot possibly be beneficial.

My three-year-old son is allergic to cow's milk and has been taking soya milk since he was six weeks old. Does he need any extra calcium and vitamins because of this? Does he need a supplement for body-building?

It will be good to give your son some Urticalcin, just to be on the safe side and to ensure that he receives sufficient calcium. Give him 2–3 tablets twice daily.

Does eating protein and carbohydrate at the same meal affect the digestion and one's health?
It is possible that this is the case. Detailed dietary guidelines can be found in my book *Nature's Gift of Food*.

If a child has a milk allergy will he or she have it for life or can it be cured?
Sometimes an allergy can be desensitised and sometimes children grow out of an allergy.

In Argyll, in past centuries, fennel was used to keep vermin away from houses. It was dried and placed on the floor, to be used like straw beds. The fennel seeds were eaten when food was scarce. The food value of fennel was nourishing and sustaining as a base for inner cleansing and a balanced foundation for digesting food. I wonder if you have ever heard about this?
Fennel is an excellent herb. I had indeed heard this story, but not from anyone who has ever practised it themselves. It is true that fennel has great cleansing properties, and fennel water is excellent when babies have problems with wind and suffer from a swollen abdomen.

When taking supplements how can we be sure that we do not disturb the balance of our immune system and the processes in our body?
Always adhere to the recommended dosage on the packaging and you cannot go wrong. It is helpful to discuss this subject with a nutritional advisor.

Could you please give us your views on compatible eating with respect to protein and carbohydrates?
This is much too complicated a subject to explain in a few words. Please read my book *Nature's Gift of Food* for advice on this subject.

I have spent considerable time changing my 'men' (husband and sons) to 'Flora men'. Is this a mistake? I thought that sunflower margarine was the healthy alternative.
Although I am not greatly in favour of margarine, Flora is acceptable. I would prefer that neither butter nor margarine was used, but a little

butter is better than margarine and butter certainly contains many more digestive enzymes.

How do you get the juice out of a raw potato?

Take a whole potato and scrub the skin properly. Grate the potato into a sieve and then press the juice out of it. Potato juice is an excellent source of alkali for controlling acidity.

My daughters, who are both vegetarian, have psoriasis. The main affected area is the scalp. Have you any suggestions for dealing with this?

They should take plenty of products rich in vitamin A. A beta carotene supplement is excellent because this is a fat-soluble substance found in green vegetables and carrots. The body is able to convert beta carotene into vitamin A, which it does according to its needs. Any beta carotene that is not converted is absorbed, circulates in the blood and is stored in fat tissues. Beta carotene is non-toxic, unlike vitamin A which can be toxic in high intakes. Therefore beta carotene is an entirely safe way to take in vitamin A, and many vegetarians rely almost solely on beta carotene for their vitamin A requirements.

However, acting as a precursor to vitamin A is by no means the only role beta carotene plays in the body. Any beta carotene that is not converted to vitamin A circulates in the blood where it acts as powerful anti-oxidant and free radical scavenger. Recently, several large-scale studies have been initiated to monitor the influence of diet on long-term health. These studies span many countries, involve hundreds of thousands of people and will last for several years. One nutrient that will be specifically focused on is beta carotene, as many nutritionists believe it may be largely responsible for the benefits of a diet high in fruit and vegetables for maintaining good health.

I have been taking Glanolin 500 (blackcurrant oil) because I have been told that it contains more gamma linolenic acid than Evening Primrose Oil. Am I doing the right thing?

I would not like to discourage you, but personally I prefer to prescribe Oil of Evening Primrose, largely because of some of the fantastic results I have seen in my patients.

Is there such a thing as a vegetarian slimming diet?

Yes, indeed. The diet I recommend to my vegetarian patients is outlined below.

Vegetarian slimming diet

Daily allowance 1 pint of skimmed milk *or* half a pint of semi-skimmed milk, *or* 2 cartons of low fat yoghurt.

Day 1 Breakfast: 1 oz cereal, a banana, tea or coffee.
Lunch: one wholemeal roll, salad and 1 oz of cheese.
Dinner: vegetable soup, a nut cutlet with curry sauce and cauliflower.

Day 2 Breakfast: tomato juice, porridge, tea or coffee.
Lunch: baked beans on toast.
Dinner: orange juice, spaghetti with tomato and mushroom sauce, salad.

Day 3 Breakfast: 1 oz cereal, an apple, tea or coffee.
Lunch: a two-egg omelette.
Dinner: filo pastry parcels, with spinach, cottage cheese, herbs and beans.

Day 4 Breakfast: V8 juice, cereal, sultanas, tea or coffee.
Lunch: fruit salad with yoghurt.
Dinner: vegetable lasagne, salad, grapes.

Day 5 Breakfast: porridge, orange juice, tea or coffee.
Lunch: mushrooms on toast.
Dinner: stuffed vine leaves with vegetable sauce, salad.

Day 6 Breakfast: cereal, orange juice, tea or coffee.
Lunch: one wholemeal roll with egg and salad, an apple.
Dinner: risotto with wild rice, vegetables and cheese sauce.

Day 7 Breakfast: muesli with nuts, tea or coffee.
Lunch: pitta bread filled with salad, 1 oz cheese.
Dinner: vegetarian pizza (small), salad.

How much codliver oil should one take?
I usually recommend one dessertspoon every evening, or one or two capsules three times daily.

I would like to know what your views are on Royal Gelee?
Royal Gelee is a wonderful gift from nature with great healing properties.

Could you please advise parents what not to include in the weekly shopping, e.g. foods that may be detrimental to teenagers in the long-term?
Primarily, I would suggest avoiding white sugar and white flour, and products that are prepared with these ingredients. Also, of course, avoid foods containing artificial flavourings, colourings and preservatives.

What are your views on the nutritional supplement Selenium ACE?
Selenium ACE is an excellent supplement because selenium is an essential mineral with several important functions in the body. It forms an integral part of the free-radical-scavenging enzyme glutathione peroxidase, which is an important natural anti-oxidant in the body. Recent research has indicated that selenium is an essential component of the enzyme that converts thyroxine into the more active tri-iodothyroxine in the thyroid gland, giving the trace mineral an important role in body metabolism.

The selenium content of food is dependent on the levels present in the soil. These levels tend to be low in Britain, presenting a problem for farmers, who often have to supplement their livestock's diets with selenium. Selenium is not added directly to deficient soil because it is not an essential trace mineral for plants and so does not feature in popular fertilisers. In addition, up to 75 per cent of selenium is lost by food refining and processing.

Honey is one of the oldest known natural foods. Many claims are made as to its healing properties. How far do you support this?
I would wholeheartedly endorse these claims. I would also always recommend the substitution of sugar with honey, because it is the best natural sweetener available to mankind.

When is it best to take vitamin pills – before or after meals?
This is usually indicated on the packaging, but if this is not stipulated, I generally recommend that supplements are taken before meals.

With the large number of additives in our food how do you suggest we obtain a balanced chemical-free diet? Inspired by one of your talks I went home and bought a juice extractor. I now take potato juice each morning and carrot juice every night – with great results.

If possible, it is always best to select organically grown produce. Juices are always good, and potato juice especially is excellent for any rheumatic disorders, eczema, and peptic, duodenal or gastric ulcers. However, let's not get too addicted to juices so that we forget to use our teeth for chewing!

Can you say which foods are energy-rich?

Fruits, vegetables, nuts and rice. In short, all natural foods contain natural energy.

How do you feel about the use of garlic oil?

Fresh garlic, garlic capsules and garlic oil – all contain good antiseptic properties and are beneficial for the immune system.

Could you please comment on not mixing carbohydrates and protein, or vegetables and fruit? I have been told that one is allowed to mix vegetables and protein, and also vegetables and carbohydrates. Is this correct?

Food-combining has become a way of life for many people. You can read about it in more detail in my book *Nature's Gift of Food*.

Where do you stand with respect to microwave cooking?

Personally, I do not use or support it because it is an unnatural way of food preparation. Food should be kept alive!

What are your views about food compatibility as advocated by 'The Hay System'?

The Hay Diet has been around for many years now and the reason it is still going strong is because it is based on a very sound nutritional foundation.

What exactly do you mean by amino acids?

Amino acids are the building blocks of protein, which are fundamental to the living cell. They may be linked together almost indefinitely to form more than 50,000 different proteins that eventually become body tissues, organs, enzymes, hormones and constituents of the immune system. Eight amino acids (although there are 22 in total) are classified as being 'essential' because the body cannot synthesise them, and these have to be obtained in adequate amounts from our food.

However, the proteins supplied in food can sometimes be difficult to break down and the process of splitting and recombining proteins is complex. Enzymes known as amino acid transferases are responsible for the interconversion between amino acids and these require vitamin B_6 which, in turn, is highly dependent on an adequate intake of protein. The effects of processing means that much 'fast food' contains relatively low levels of vitamin B_6 compared with its protein content.

The number and level of essential amino acids in foods determines the quality of the protein. Most animal proteins contain all eight essential amino acids, whereas single vegetable proteins are 'incomplete' proteins and may not contain all the essential amino acids. Vegetarians and vegans often choose to supplement their intake of protein. Free-form amino acid supplements supply protein that is already conveniently broken down into its building blocks, so that it can be easily assimilated. These supplements could be useful during periods of illness and convalescence, in old age, or at difficult times when food preparation and therefore its digestion may suffer.

Do you know where I can buy good hawthornberry jam? I understand they sell it in Europe.
Yes, hawthornberry jam is readily available on the mainland of Europe, but what is to stop you making it yourself?

What dosage would you recommend for Primrose Oil capsules?
Unless there are unusual circumstances I usually prescribe three 500 mg capsules to be taken at night before going to bed.

What are the five foods to eliminate from the diet when suffering from _Candida_ problems?
Wine, cheese, sugar (including chocolate), fermented foods (i.e. yeast products) and mushrooms should all be eliminated from the diet.

Should amino acids be taken in combination or individually?
They can be taken either way; the choice depends largely upon the formula and upon the individual circumstances and requirements.

How do you feel about young children being given fluoride supplements and fluoride coating on their teeth?
This, fortunately, is the individual choice of the parents, rather than imposed self-medication in the drinking water.

Should Evening Primrose Oil be used internally or externally for the healing and/or removal of scars?
External use of Evening Primrose Oil is ideal for promoting the healing of scars and wounds.

Should vitamin C tablets be taken when citrus fruits have been vetoed?
Yes, these tablets are not detrimental to certain conditions in the same way as citrus fruits. Take at least 1 or 2 g per day.

How do you feel about *Acidophilus* and *Biodophilus* taken in combination, or should they be taken separately?
Either supplement is excellent, but I would prefer to see them taken separately.

Would you please give me the name of Dr Vogel's calcium preparation which can be easily absorbed by the body?
The excellent preparation you refer to is known as Urticalcin.

Can you please advise me on macrobiotic diets? I have been following such a regime for the past six weeks and am finding it helpful (I have ME). Would there by any long-term problems?
Macrobiotic diets should be followed to the letter and it is advisable to do so under medical supervision.

Is it necessary to take vitamin, mineral and herbal supplements on a daily basis?
If the quality of your food is adequate, i.e. if it is organically grown and correctly prepared, there is no need. However, few diets fulfil these requirements and therefore in many cases a daily supplement is required.

It seems rather an inadequate explanation for doctors to say that heredity governs the intake of nutrients from food by

our bodies. What can be changed?

Consult a dietician or good nutritional counsellor for further advice.

Recently I have read about fruit and vegetables receiving a blast of radiation to increase their shelf storage time. What are your views on this?

I am very much against it and prefer my fruit and vegetables organically grown. You can read more about this subject in my book *Nature's Gift of Food*.

While I agree that diet does play a very important part in the health of a person, I also feel that their mental attitude is very important. What do you think?

I totally agree with you. A positive mind is often the best cure.

Does cider vinegar taken in a little water every day have any health benefits?

For rheumatism or rheumatic complaints the potassium in the cider vinegar is definitely beneficial. I would not suggest that you take this remedy continuously over a long period, because the body will benefit more if the programme is stopped for a while.

Do you think microwave ovens are safe – healthwise – if used for many years, or might there be a danger to the health of people using them on a regular basis?

I am not in favour of using microwave ovens for the preparation of food. If it is absolutely necessary, use them with common sense.

Is there an alternative to using butter when quickly frying vegetables or Tofu? I first dip Tofu in a crumbled mixture of cornmeal and vegetarian chicken seasoning and brown it. I cannot get this result with water. Is there another way? Since Tofu and fish are my only source of protein, I use this method frequently and worry about the harm I may be doing. Fish is not a problem as I can poach it, but Tofu is flavourless when prepared in water.

Why not use sunflower or vegetable oil? Often olive oil is good too!

Where can I buy Molkosan?

Molkosan is a natural whey product and can be obtained from most healthfood stores, chemists or from Bioforce (the address can be found on page 280).

I understand that chromium is supposed to be beneficial. Can you please tell me from which natural source it is derived?

Chromium is excellent because it is an essential component of a substance called GTF (glucose tolerance factor), a compound made up of vitamin B_3 and a trio of amino acids. It assists in the action of insulin by enabling the cells to take up glucose for energy release and probably helps in the synthesis of fatty acids and cholesterol.

Our supply of the blood-sugar-balancing mineral chromium is sometimes low because of difficulties in breaking down the form in which it is supplied, which is mainly from meat and shellfish. Food processing and agricultural methods also tend to deplete our dietary intake of chromium. Chromium is not an essential mineral for plants, so modern synthetic fertilisers do not contain it.

The body's supplies of chromium decrease as we age and researchers now suggest that this may also happen when poor dietary habits do not replace the chromium which the body is slowly using up. Vegetarians and vegans may choose to supplement their diet with this trace mineral. Women who are pregnant also often choose to take a chromium supplement, on their doctor's advice.

What about cell salts – do you recommend them?

Cell tissue salts are excellent for many different purposes.

Do you recommend milk products for general use?

I would always be wary of the indiscriminate and excessive use of dairy foods. Use them in moderation, e.g. no more than half a pint of milk per day. Yoghurt and cottage cheese are exceptions to this rule.

Could you please give me your thoughts, please, on the value of eating meat, fish or chicken?

Meat and poultry are sources of protein and fat but, unlike vegetables, they are a 'dead' food. In naturopathic medicine food of vegetable origin is considered to contain a certain 'life energy' which is conducive to health. Fish provides a good supply of protein, as well as a number of amino acids which are beneficial for certain medical conditions.

How do you feel about including an oil cure in a diet for arthritis and how should one go about it?

In answer to your question I quote below from a programme on the codliver oil course, which has benefited many people with arthritic complaints:

1. Eliminate 'synthetic' foods – all processed, preservative-added or valueless foods or snacks. Include plenty of fresh vegetables, fish, fresh fruits and eat less meat.

2. Add codliver oil to your diet. It may be of real benefit because it helps to lubricate the tissues surrounding the joints. Dryness in the linings of the joints is the main obstacle to be overcome. Taking capsules of codliver oil is not going to be effective for this purpose. Capsules are made out of gelatin which affects the digestion and sends the codliver oil to the liver. This does very little to lubricate the joints.

3. Keep painkillers to a minimum. Users of aspirin and cortisone will attest to the fact that these drugs are not a cure. Menopausal women taking cortisone may find their faces ballooning and experience increased hot flushes and a rise in their blood pressure. Let your body produce its own cortisone. Your adrenal glands can do this if there is enough vitamin D in the body. Codliver oil, if it is emulsified, can send oil bubbles containing vitamin D to your adrenal glands. Cortisone made in this way is more sticky and may increase the consistency of the collagen in your body, which supports bone, cartilage, ligaments, tendons and other connective tissue. When you create your own cortisone, you add viscosity to your collagen, so that the oils will be held in place near your joints.

4. If you drink tea or coffee, drink it ten minutes before a meal, not with or after your meals. Of course, it would be healthier to avoid these beverages altogether. Herbal teas or coffee substitutes are more healthy choices. (The tannic acid in tea dries out the linings of the joints; caffeine also has a drying effect.)

5. Carbonated beverages should be avoided, in view of the chemicals, artificial colourings and flavourings and excess sugar they contain.

6. Allergies can be a warning sign of impending arthritis, so it makes sense to avoid foods that trigger allergic responses.

7. Chew acid fruits to neutralise them. Don't bypass your saliva by drinking juice concentrates or they will make your body too acidic. Your body will only heal in an alkaline state. To neutralise acids, your body robs mineral salts from your blood and tissues, which encourages degeneration and resulting arthritis. Your saliva can help to combat these acids, so chew everything very well.

8. Supplement your diet with vitamins B, C and E, and the minerals zinc and manganese, as these nutrients are often deficient in our food.

9. Using ice cubes in your drinks quickly congeals your dietary oils, so all nutritive value to your joints is lost.

10. Drink liquids ten minutes before or four hours after eating, to allow the oils to be assimilated properly.

11. Make sure your bowels are moving adequately (two or three times daily).

12. Avoid microwaved food. The high temperature incinerates your food, burning away enzymes and minerals.

Does bread with more than one grain, e.g. wheat and rye, constitute incorrect food-combining?

No, this is not an incorrect combination, both components belong to the grain family.

Given a choice, would you select a bread made with yeast or without it?

Sourdough bread is the best choice. There are so many people with *Candida* and yeast has a detrimental influence on this condition.

I read recently that some gum disease is caused by calcium deficiency. The remedy recommended was bonemeal. Can you say what daily intake would be necessary?

One cannot generalise on this subject, because there could be many other reasons for gum disease. If you have decided that bonemeal is what you would like to take, follow the instructions given on the packaging.

What foods should I avoid as I have a hiatus hernia?
Specifically, fatty and highly acid foods should be banned from your diet.

What foods should I eat (apart from bananas) to maintain a high level of potassium?
Foods rich in potassium are bananas, potatoes, apricots, dates, cider vinegar, molasses and dried fruits.

Would giving up red meat completely do me any harm?
No, not in the slightest, because the body can do very well without it.

I have heard about the benefits of artichokes. How would you suggest preparing them?
Jerusalem artichokes especially are very good for liver cleansing. They can be cooked in a little water (like most other vegetables), or used for soup, and they can even be fried in a little sunflower oil. The choice depends on your personal preference.

I have been attending a herbalist as I suffered from dizzy attacks. I was advised to take herbal medicine and that I shouldn't eat anything from the pig, nor dairy products. I have been following a dairy-free diet, but could you tell me why I shouldn't eat anything from a pig?
Pork has the highest content of animal fat and animal acid of any meat. You were well advised to avoid pork in any shape or form.

Can honey be used as a direct substitute for sugar, or are molasses better?
Both are natural products and you may use either according to personal preferences.

When substituting for cow's milk, is it better to use goat's milk or soya milk?
Both are acceptable, but in cases of allergies soya is usually preferred.

What vitamin or mineral supplement would you recommend for someone on a wholefood diet?
Preferably, I would suggest something that is of particular help to a poor digestive system. Health Insurance Plus is an excellent combination supplement for this purpose.

There is much concern over the dosing of babies and small children with fluoride tablets and drops. What are your thoughts?
I would prefer to see the diet adapted in such a way that no supplementary fluoride is required. Children should be given plenty of fresh fruit and vegetables, especially carrots.

Can we improve the soil in our garden vegetable plot with regard to its zinc and potassium content?
Avoid the use of herbicides, pesticides and artificial fertilisers. Use natural products for the purpose of fertilisation.

Does a person on a vegetarian diet need extra vitamins?
Vegetarians should always include plenty of nuts in their diet, and it is worth remembering that nearly everyone nowadays is in need of a vitamin supplement occasionally.

What do you think of the soya bean as a source of protein?
The soya bean is the best possible source of protein. Fortunately, it is widely grown the world over and is readily available to the populations of poorer nations as well.

I have been told that vitamin C is very good. I use it to keep clear of colds. I drink a lot of milk. I am 92 years old. How much should I use?
Congratulations on your age! It pays to invest in your health. I would suggest that you take about 1 g of vitamin C a day and you will be safe.

Why is alternative medicine not called original medicine? It was here long before orthodox medicine.
A good idea – but it's too late now to turn the clock back!

For how long should herbal cures be taken? Should the body not have a break from them every now and then?

You are quite right, long-term indiscriminate use will make certain substances less efficient.

203

O

OVARIES

Is there a suitable remedy for the treatment of inflamed ovaries?
Apis mellifica is the best remedy for inflamed ovaries. Please consult a qualified practitioner who will advise you.

I have had surgery for ovarian cysts and would like to know if homoeopathy could help, either instead of, or as well as, surgery?
Use the homoeopathic remedy *Ovarium* or Ovasan and see if that will help you to keep the condition under control.

P

PERSPIRATION

What would you advise for excessive perspiration?
Take 15 drops of *Menosan* twice daily.

What can I do for excessive sweating of the feet?
Before going to bed at night wash the feet thoroughly and then rub in zinc and caster oil cream, which is readily available from most chemists. Cover the feet with an old pair of cotton socks to avoid staining the bed clothes. Keep this up for a few weeks and after that you may only have to do this once a week, or as required.

Because I suffer so badly from sweaty feet I am very hard on my shoes. What can I do about it?
Sprinkle some borax into the shoes every day. You will find that you will soon only have to do this once a week or so, and after that only occasionally.

PHLEBITIS

What is phlebitis?
Phlebitis is the name for an inflammation of a vein or veins. Usually a large vein is involved. The condition is mostly associated with varicose veins.

Is there a remedy for phlebitis?
Witch hazel will often be helpful. Take 15 drops of *Hamamelis virg.* (a witch hazel extract) twice daily.

PREGNANCY

I have two children and at both births I have had a very long and difficult labour. I am now pregnant again and I wonder if you would have any suggestions?
Before the baby is due take 10 drops of *Aesculus hipp.* (horse chestnut extract) twice daily.

Is there any harm in taking Oil of Evening Primrose while breast feeding?
Please do not worry, because there is no harm in lactating mothers taking Oil of Evening Primrose.

Is there a natural herb for birth control?
I must disappoint you in this respect. Although there are some herbs that are supposed to reduce fertility, nature does not seem to have supplied us with a reliable herb for this purpose.

I read the book *Wild Yam Birth Control Without Fear.* Have you heard about it and if so, do you believe this method is effective?
Wild yams have been used by some indigenous peoples for the purpose of birth control, but I would not rely on them!

What advice would you give a newly pregnant mother-to-be to ensure a safe and happy pregnancy? Is there *one* golden rule?
I designed the following programme many years ago and many of my patients have happily followed it:

Homoeopathic pregnancy package

1. *Caulophyllum 30:* Take two doses, morning and evening, on alternate days, commencing two months prior to delivery date.

2. *Arnica 30:* This remedy may be used at any time throughout pregnancy for the relief of soreness, tiredness and stretching of tissues, but should be taken daily for two weeks prior to delivery.

3. *Bellis perennis 12x:* Following delivery, take one powder daily for four doses, together with one dose daily of *Arnica 30.*

4. Calendula Mother Tincture: Twelve drops in a cup of warm, sterile water is useful for swabbing the perineal area after delivery.

5. Calendula ointment: This will assist healing if smeared lightly on any irritation.

N.B. Suck or chew capsules or tablets between meals – they should not be swallowed with water. Tip the dose onto the lid of the bottle and transfer to the mouth. Similarly, the powders should be placed directly on the tongue and allowed to dissolve in the mouth – no water should be taken.

Vitamin/mineral supplements recommended during pregnancy

Months 1–3:   B50 Complex, folic acid 400 mcg, vitamin C 500 mg with bioflavanoids.

Months 4 and 5:   Vitamin E 200 IU, vitamin C 500 mg with bioflavanoids, multivitamin/mineral capsule, molasses capsule.

Month 6:   B50 Complex, vitamin C 500 mg with bioflavanoids, vitamin E 200 IU, multi-chelated mineral tablet, molasses capsules.

Month 7 onward: Same as for months 4 and 5.

I am pregnant and have constant nausea. Is there a safe remedy?
Take ten drops of *Nux vomica D3* twice daily.

PROSTATE PROBLEMS

Is there anything you can advise for prostate problems? My husband does not want an operation and I am nearly round the bend with him.
Fortunately, I can reassure you, because at last a very good product has become available: Prostabrit. This product is imported from Denmark and many of my patients have already confirmed its efficacy. As prostate

problems are much more common than is generally thought, but because of their nature are cloaked in a certain amount of secrecy, I will go into some detail here.

More than 30,000 prostatectomies are carried out in the UK each year. In the USA this figure is ten times as high. The cost to the National Health Service is about one hundred million pounds per annum. Three-quarters of men over the age of 50 in the UK have some non-cancerous enlargement of their prostate gland. More than a third of a million go to their GP for help, yet many more suffer it in silence. Ninety per cent of all men over the age of 65 have a non-cancerous enlargment of their prostate and between a third and half have urinary symptoms that make them seek medical help. Eventually, about three-quarters of men will need some sort of treatment for prostate enlargement. This represents an epidemic by any standard. If such a condition affected women, there would be a public outcry.

The prostate is a reproductive and sexual gland which lies in the base of the bladder in men, surrounding the part of the urinary passage that carries urine from the bladder to the penis. At birth it is about the size of a pea and it gradually enlarges until puberty, when it grows to the size of a walnut. A normal healthy prostate gland weighs up to 20 g.

Why men have a prostate is not fully understood. What we do know is that it is made up of millions of tiny glands, as well as muscle and fibrous tissue. The main function of the prostate is to secrete nutritious fluids required for the transportation of healthy semen. Prostabrit is a dietary supplement specifically designed for the purpose of containing and overcoming prostate irregularities. This supplement is available from larger chemists and health stores and comes accompanied by very useful dietary suggestions.

Is there a natural remedy for an enlarged prostate gland as an alternative to a surgical operation? Presently I take two Indoramin tablets per day, resulting in a minor improvement in the condition.
Try Prostabrit.

I know that I have prostate problems because of constant urges to urinate, but I also have shooting pains. Can you advise me?
Take Prostabrit, but for the pains I would recommend that you also take 15 drops of Prostasan twice daily.

Can you advise on how to prevent prostate gland problems?
Every day chew two tablespoons of pumpkin seeds, either roasted or fresh. A little zinc will also help and Nature's Best's Zinc Citrate is a useful supplement because it has been specifically designed for more efficient absorption and better use by the body. Zinc Citrate bonds the trace elements to a key substance used in energy metabolism. This form of zinc is easily assimilated and is therefore very useful for people with a slightly sensitive digestive system.

What can be done for an enlarged prostate, i.e. three times its normal size? I am taking the herb saw palmetto, but it does not seem to be helping much.
Saw palmetto is a good remedy, but considering the severity of the problem I would suggest that you start taking Prostabrit, together with Zinc Citrate.

What to do about calcium deposits in the urinary tract, complicated by an inflamed prostate gland?
Start using Urticalcin, which will be absorbed and not amass into deposits in the body. Also take Prostabrit.

I have been told by my GP that I have prostatitis and his solution was to prescribe a course of antibiotics. Can you advise if there are any natural remedies?
There is a very good remedy called Prostasan in the Bioforce range – take ten drops three times daily.

I have prostate problems and need to pass water frequently – also during the night. What can I do to get a good night's sleep?
I am sure that Prostabrit will help.

PSORIASIS

My daughter has psoriasis and wants to know about any alternative treatment possibilities. Can you advise her?
I have written two books on the subject and she can perhaps borrow these from her local library and read up on it. The books are *Skin Disorders* and *Arthritis, Rheumatism and Psoriasis*.

Is it really possible to contain – or better, to overcome – psoriasis?

It must be understood that psoriasis can be cured, but only from the inside. There is no use in putting on layers of ointments unless the healing has started internally. Therefore diet is very important. The main dietary guidelines here are to avoid pork in any shape or form, cut out citrus fruits, use salt and spices sparingly and avoid alcohol and chocolate. For more detailed information please read my books, as mentioned above.

Is it wise to take zinc tablets to help with psoriasis?

Supplementary zinc is indeed helpful, but is insufficient on its own. Oil of Evening Primrose should also be taken and, dependent upon your condition, there are other herbal remedies that may be useful.

My son is 30 years old and has suffered for a number of years with psoriasis. Although he attends a homoeopathic practitioner he does not seem to be improving. Do you have any suggestions please?

In persistent cases I have successfully prescribed a Japanese remedy called *Perilla* extract. Usually I recommend that the patient takes this in combination with the Formula ECZ, and the results have been most encouraging.

Can you suggest anything that will help for chronic psoriasis?

A well-balanced diet, herbal remedies (see my book *Skin Disorders*) and plenty of exercise in the fresh air are all beneficial.

What is the cause of psoriasis and what are the alternative treatments?

Sometimes this condition is the result of an inherited factor where the epidermis produces new cells before keratin formation has taken place. There are many forms of alternative treatment and I would suggest that you read my book *Skin Disorders* for further details.

My son suffers from psoriasis. It seems to run in the family and it flares up at certain times of the year, especially on his knees and joints. He is going on holiday soon and would like to know if you can help?

There are many forms of psoriasis and, as you have already noted, the condition can run in the family. When your son goes on holiday suggest that he takes every opportunity to catch some sunshine; bathing in sea water is also very good for psoriasis. You should also discuss possible diets with him, according to the guidelines found in the books mentioned above.

Please tell me something about psoriasis and what is the name of the internal cleansing treatment?

In answer to the first part of your question, please refer to the rest of this section. With regard to your second query, the Dr Vogel Detox Box Programme will make an excellent start to any treatment. It contains five natural remedies and detailed dietary advice.

I am bothered with psoriasis and for the last two years I have been plagued by sore toes. I have tried sulphur tablets and Oil of Evening Primrose capsules. Do you have any other suggestions?

You are on the right road, but I would suggest that you also use *Perilla* extract internally and dab the toes with *Spilanthes*.

My husband is aged 31 and has ankylosing spondylitis and psoriasis. What would you suggest for him?

Try to get him to follow the programme known as the Detox Box Programme, which is available from Bioforce. Also, please read my book *Arthritis, Rheumatism and Psoriasis* for advice on both conditions, because his illnesses are often interlinked.

I am 55 years old and suffer from psoriasis. The pads of my toes are very sore and I wonder if you have any suggestions?

Rub Symphytum onto the affected areas, or dab on *Spilanthen*. Either remedy has proved very useful in cases similar to yours.

How long must I wait to see the results of a detoxification and macrobiotic diet for psoriasis? I know that it usually gets worse before it gets better, but can you give me an idea of the time involved?

You are quite right, because usually the condition seems to deteriorate before any signs of improvement are noticeable. That is how natural medicine works, particularly while the body is being detoxified. It is impossible to give you a definite time-scale.

R

RESTLESS LEGS

What can be done about restless legs? Often when I lie in bed I have to get up because of the intense discomfort in my legs, causing an all-over feeling of restlessness.

Take twice daily one capsule of vitamin E d-alpha tocopherol, because vitamin E in its natural form is d-alpha tocopherol. This is the form in which vitamin E occurs in foodstuffs and our bodies are able to absorb tocopherol very efficiently. In fact, when vitamin E is supplied as d-alpha tocopheryl acetate (commonly used in supplements), the body has to first remove the acetate part of the molecule and this is carried out by the enzymes of the digestive system. Only when the tocopherol is released by this enzyme action can it be absorbed into the blood stream.

My mother-in-law has restless legs that keep twitching. She has tried magnesium without any success.

Sometimes magnesium orotate helps, but always use vitamin E at the same time.

Sometimes I cannot keep my legs still at night. Can you tell me what causes this?

Restless legs can be due to drinking too much tea or coffee, but it can also be caused by a vitamin deficiency. Please take 400–500 IU of vitamin E twice daily and for extra help you may like to take 5 mg of Folic Acid, also twice daily.

RHEUMATISM

(*see* ARTHRITIS AND RHEUMATISM)

S

SCHIZOPHRENIA

I have a schizophrenic son and would like to have your advice.
Most schizophrenics are allergic to sugar. Ban sugar altogether from the diet and read my book *Multiple Sclerosis* for details of the Roger McDougall diet. Although this diet is largely promoted for MS patients, I have also seen some very good results in patients with schizophrenia who have followed it.

Are there any alternative remedies that are suitable for the treatment of mental illnesses, i.e. schizoprehnia?
There are indeed some homoeopathic remedies for the treatment of schizophrenia, but I hasten to add that such treatment should always take place under the guidance of a qualified homoeopathic practitioner. Self-help is possible, however, if you concentrate on the nutritional approach. I would suggest supplementary vitamin B complex, vitamin C, zinc, selenium and manganese.

Could you please give me some advice on mental illness, especially schizophrenia and the awful depression that it causes.
Depression is always the most difficult part of the illness for a schizophrenic to bear. From experience in my practice, I would suggest using zinc, Valerian and *Cerebrum*. I must repeat that the treatment in such cases should take place under medical supervision, when the patient's exact requirements can be worked out.

How would an alternative practitioner treat schizophrenia?
Depending on the individual patient, a practitioner could choose to apply

acupuncture, colour therapy or dietary management, together with herbal and homoeopathic remedies.

Can you tell me more about food patterns for schizophrenics? I live with one.
Living with a schizophrenic requires a great deal of patience and understanding. Substances to avoid are sugar, chocolate, alcohol, nicotine, coffee and salt, etc. Again, I would suggest that you study the gluten-free diet outlined in my book *Multiple Sclerosis*.

Can you help me – I am a female schizophrenic aged 34?
Read the answers to previous questions on this topic and pay particular attention to the dietary instructions. I must also emphasise that it would be worth your while consulting a homoeopathic practitioner, who may be able to help you.

SCIATICA

Could you please explain exactly what sciatica is?
Fortunately, sciatica is not anywhere near as common as is generally believed. Too often, certain back or lower back pains are referred to as sciatica. True sciatica is brought about by compression of a disc on the sciatic nerve, which is the longest nerve in the body, and only in cases of a prolapse of the intervertebral disc or its protrusion on the nerve root should the term sciatica be used. This condition can indeed be the cause of a most excruciating pain. I mostly apply acupuncture or laser treatment to sciatica patients, and recommend Imperthritica for the inflammation. Some patients also react well to *Arnica*.

What homoeopathic remedies or treatment methods can be used for sciatica?
I would suggest either one of the homoeopathic remedies *Gelsemium* or *Symphytum*.

SHINGLES (*Herpes zoster*)

What can be done for shingles?
Shingles is caused by an extremely persistent and nasty virus. This virus is

the same one that causes chickenpox; it may lie dormant in the nerve root and can be activated by stress. Suitable homoeopathic remedies are *Merzerium, Rhus tox, Lachesis* and *Avena sativa.* It is interesting to know that the best results my patients have reported back to me were obtained when the American remedy ViraPlex was used, available from Enzymatic Therapy.

What can be taken for *Herpes zoster* externally?
Touch the affected areas every day with a leek that has been sliced open. Better still, put some leeks through a juice extractor and dab the skin with the juice.

Is there a cure for *Herpes zoster*?
I couldn't go so far as to claim that *Herpes zoster* can be cured. It would be better to say that it is possible to keep this condition under control. I would advise 15 drops of *Avena sativa* taken twice daily together with two ViraPlex tablets.

I have had shingles all over my face, but fortunately it has mostly cleared up. I am now left with a very stubborn inflamed patch which I do not seem able to shift. I am allergic to lanolin and Vaseline and wonder if you could advise anything else to relieve this.
With shingles great care should always be taken not to touch the affected patches with soap and water. For soap, please also read both foams and shower gels. It is best to leave these inflamed patches alone, even though you may not feel very good about them. This condition can only be cleared from the inside. The only external treatment I would suggest is dabbing with leek juice, even though the smell may be somewhat off-putting.

Please advise me on how shingles may be helped.
As a major contributory factor to shingles is stress, I often advise patients to follow a low stress diet. Guidelines for such a diet can be found in my book *Stress and Nervous Disorders.* Also, various homoeopathic remedies may be taken, as mentioned above and I would stress that you take action as soon as possible to avoid this condition really establishing itself.

My husband has had shingles for two weeks and he has used the lotion given to him by the doctor for four days. Now he is on painkillers. He is getting very little sleep. He is 71 years

old and takes vitamins B and C, Selenium ACE and
multivitamins. Is there anything he can take to relieve the
pain and allow him some sleep?

He is following a very sensible programme, but considering the present
circumstances I would add *Merzerium* (ten drops, twice daily) and two
tablets of ViraPlex.

My mother has shingles and is being discharged from
hospital. She is taking cortisone, but is there a natural
alternative she could take?

I would not substitute the cortisone, but as well as cortisone I would also
give her 15 drops of *Avena sativa* together with three Urticalcin tablets to
be taken twice daily before meals. Twice daily after meals give her one
ViraPlex tablet.

SINUSITIS

I have a persistent frontal sinusitis that will not clear. What
would you advise?

Over the years many of my patients have sung the praises of the Sinus
Formula available from Bioforce. Take 15 drops twice a day, together with
Cinnabaris 3x three tablets, also twice daily. With regard to your diet, cut
out all dairy foods and salt and eat extra garlic and plenty of honey.

I suffer badly from sinus problems which cause head pains as
well as face pains. Are there any suitable homoeopathic
remedies?

Applicable homoeopathic remedies are *Cinnabaris 3x, Kal. chlor. 6x, Nat.
mur. 6x,* and *Belladonna 30x.*

My eight-year-old daughter keeps getting sinusitis. What
remedy would you suggest?

Give her ten drops of Formula SNS twice daily and watch her diet: limit
her intake of dairy food and salt.

I have had sinus problems for 12 months and would like to
know if you could help me?

This problem can be very persistent and I know people who have had sinus complaints for many years. Take Sinus Formula, cut out all dairy foods and start immediately on a salt-free diet.

I am greatly troubled by sinusitis and catarrh. What can you recommend?

These ailments often go hand in hand. Cut out dairy foods, start on a salt-free diet and take Sinus Formula for the sinusitis and Echinaforce for the catarrh.

Please advise me on sinus problems with severe headaches.

If the headaches are bad take SinuCheck from Enzymatic Therapy. Also follow the dietary restrictions as mentioned above.

Does horseradish cure sinus congestion? If not, what does?

Horseradish helps greatly, but it will not clear up the condition without some extra help. Also take *Cinnabaris 3x* and take extra garlic.

I have been given three weeks' supply of very powerful antibiotics to combat chronic sinusitis. Is there another way to combat chronic problems like this?

Antibiotics are rarely capable of overcoming or clearing sinusitis. Unless you follow the dietary advice given elsewhere in this section there is very little chance of the condition improving.

What would you prescribe for a lady with very bad sinusitis? She is overweight – does that have any connection?

Carrying too much weight is never good for one's health. I wouldn't go so far as to agree that there is a connection, but it can only be helpful if that lady sheds some of her excess weight. She should cut out dairy foods, sugar and salt, and see what happens.

My son has sinus problems. The doctors want to take out his adenoids because he also breathes very heavily. Do you agree?

Sometimes, when the sinuses are inflamed, the adenoids also become swollen. If that is the case with your son I would suggest you give him 15 drops of *Marum verum* twice daily.

What can I do for sinus problems and allergies?

Allergic reactions, especially to dairy foods, play a large role in sinus conditions. However, other allergies may be involved and I suggest that you ask your doctor for some tests.

How would you help an acute attack of tonsillitis and sinusitis, which is most painful, particularly the sinusitis?

The best approach would be to take Sinu-Check, which will take the pain away.

Please can you advise me on sinus problems. I have had antibiotics for sinus problems, but get very bad headaches which stop me being able to concentrate. I have thought of going to see an acupuncturist, but I don't know if this would be useful. I am also slightly worried at the thought of needles.

Acupuncture treatment would certainly be a very wise move. You would be surprised at the number of people who share your concern about visiting an acupuncturist. However, there is absolutely no reason to be afraid. The needles are practically painless and any qualified acupuncturist will do his or her best to reassure you.

Could you recommend suitable remedies for chronic colds and sinusitis?

Take 15 drops of Echinaforce three times a day and four tablets of Urticalcin twice a day.

Can you please explain if there is a link between allergies and sinus problems?

Most allergic problems occur when the immune system is under pressure. I am sure that if you took a course of Imuno-Strength you would benefit. The immune system is distributed throughout the body and is composed of white cells found in the lymph glands, liver, spleen, blood and bone marrow.

There are two main types of white cells: granulocytes, which produce an immediate response to a challenge by releasing chemicals, and lymphocytes, which produce a delayed response, adjusting their attack to the new invader, or remembering it from a previous time. There are two types of lymphocytes: B-cells which produce antibodies and T-cells that modify this response.

The components of the immune system described briefly above rely on the nutrients in our diet for their production and maintenance. For example, zinc is included in the Imuno-Strength preparation since the thymus gland, which produces T-cells, requires this nutrient for its healthy functioning. Also included are two herbs which have been associated with the immune system for centuries: *Echinacea purpurea*, or the coneflower, which is widely cultivated for its gorgeous flowers and which has been extensively analysed to identify its active compounds, and Devil's Claw, an African plant bearing large, hooked claw-like fruits, which is currently receiving a great deal of publicity for its reported benefits.

It is essential to maintain a healthy immune system, and an important step towards this is to ensure that the system receives the nutritional support that it needs. Imuno-Strength can help safeguard the supply of important nutrients when the diet is not all that it should be.

SKIN DISORDERS

I often experience itching all over my body, which makes me extremely irritable and difficult to live with. What can I do?
This condition can often be cleared by a liver-cleansing programme. Consider following the recommended dietary instructions outlined on pages 150-1.

I suffer from *Lichen planus* and would be grateful if you could suggest something to ease the itching, especially at night.
Lichen planus manifests itself as an outbreak of tiny purple or red lumps, mostly on the arms and legs. It can also affect the scalp and can cause hair loss or nail deformities. It can be treated by *Sulphur 6x* and *Rumis 6x*, and in the case of burning sensations you should try *Arsenicum 6x*. In all cases taking 15 drops of Echinaforce twice daily will be beneficial.

I have had a skin rash – *Lichen planus* – for six years. At the hospital they say that they cannot do anything. Have you any suggestions?
Use the remedies suggested in response to the above question and also take good care of your diet. For general advice please read my book *Skin Disorders*.

I have had *Pityriasis rubra pilaris* (a skin condition) for one year. I have taken Etrenate capsules, bathed with oil and used an emulsifying ointment. Apparently, it takes two years to clear the condition out of the system and it also causes liver damage and hair loss. Please could you tell me what caused this condition as the skin specialist would not or cannot tell me. Is there anything I can take to clear up the last few patches?

This condition is generally thought to be caused by a virus. To clear the remaining patches take three 500 mg capsules of Oil of Evening Primrose before going to bed. Also take, twice daily, ten drops of Petaforce after meals in half a cup of water.

I have an irritation on the lower part of the leg which I try not to scratch. When I do I tear the skin and scratch until the leg bleeds. It started as an irritating little red spot that spread to a rash.

Dab the affected area with cider vinegar or with leek juice. Yet another option is to use Molkosan for external treatment.

My wife, aged 54, has suffered from rosacea on her face for the past five years. It can be controlled with antibiotics, but she doesn't want to take them for the rest of her life. She has been to a homoeopathic doctor who could not help and is now seeing another, who attributes the problem to stress.

The condition is very often associated with emotions and stress, although it is sometimes due to a deficiency of vitamin B_2. Fortunately, there are alternative treatment methods to antibiotics and I often use acupuncture and naturopathic remedies such as *Lachesis 6x, Nux vomica 3x* and *Sulph. iod. 6x*, and as a highly effective herbal antibiotic I mostly prescribe Echinaforce.

I am in my late forties and I have developed a rash down one side of my face – on my eyelids and the side of my mouth. I have heard that this can be a menopausal symptom. Is this correct?

The hormonal imbalance during the menopause can indeed cause conditions such as you describe. Take Oil of Evening Primrose (three capsules before going to bed) and also 20 drops of Echinaforce twice daily.

I have a constant fine rash, which at times flares up like big welts. What would you advise?
Use Dr Vogel's 7 Herb Cream and take 15 drops of Echinaforce twice daily.

I have used a cortisone cream for 26 years for localised dermatitis. What could the effects of this cream be and what should I do to treat my skin holistically?
It would be better if you could manage to stop using the cortisone cream. The holistic approach would include diet, herbal ointments, homoeopathic and herbal remedies. For further details please read my book *Skin Disorders*.

For over a year I have had constant itching on my back. It is not a dermatological problem. What could be wrong?
Consult a qualified practitioner for an accurate diagnosis. Meanwhile, use some *Sulphur 3x* and wash your back with a soap substitute that does not contain soap.

I have a ten-year-old daughter who has very dry skin and I have been giving her Evening Primrose Oil to help. Now I have heard that this is no good if someone suffers from epilepsy, which my daughter did when she was younger.
Indeed, you had better not give her Oil of Evening Primrose. Why not substitute this by using olive oil in your cooking and continue to watch her diet carefully?

I stopped smoking four years ago, since when I have experienced weight gain and loss of skin pigmentation. Is there any connection?
Not really. The weight gain should only be temporary, as this is a common complaint when people first give up smoking, but this should have settled by now. I suggest that you take three 500 mg capsules of Oil of Evening Primrose at night.

What can be done for a child troubled with cracking skin caused by a fungus?
Dab the affected areas with *Spilanthes*.

Is there a non-surgical means of removing old scar tissue, e.g. from severe burns in childhood?
I use cosmetic acupuncture and Oil of Evening Primrose in such cases.

Can anything be done for brown pigmentation spots which appear with ageing?
Follow the liver diet as outlined on pages 150-1. Also use *Chelidonium* (ten drops, twice daily).

What causes puffiness under the eyes?
This sometimes indicates an irregularity in the kidney function. You may be wise to have this investigated.

What can be done about moles, or skin spots that are sometimes also called liver spots?
Follow the liver diet (see pages 150-1).

Every now and then I develop a rash on my legs and have had this complaint for approximately eight or ten years. (My father has the same thing.) Nothing seems to help. Some dermatologists say that it is psoriasis and others do not know what it is. What should I do?
This sounds as if the diagnosis of psoriasis may be correct. Read both my books *Skin Disorders* and *Arthritis, Rheumatism and Psoriasis* for further advice.

Are there any plants that can be used topically to help lighten moles or freckles? In an article on homoeopathy I read that *Cantharis* may help.
Some practitioners may indeed prescribe *Cantharis* for the purpose you refer to.

I have cysts on my scalp. Is there anything I can do?
Take ten drops of Petaforce after meals, twice daily.

What is required for beautiful skin?
Apart from the fact that the quality of skin is often determined by hereditary factors, diet is also extremely important. Eat plenty of vegetables and fruits and take the essential oils. Cleanse the skin well and

care for it sensibly. Additional general advice can be found in my book *Skin Disorders*.

My sister, who is now 53 years old, has always suffered from dry, rough and scaly skin on her arms, legs and back. Do you know of anything which would help her condition?
Advise her to cook with olive oil and suggest that she take three 500 mg capsules of Oil of Evening Primrose at night.

What is the cause of discoloration of the skin?
Such conditions are usually caused by deficiencies of vitamins, minerals and trace elements. Please try a balanced supplement, e.g Health Insurance Plus.

I get skin rashes from sunlight. Can anything be done?
Some people are allergic to sunlight, so please be careful. There are remedies that can help but, unfortunately, I cannot advise you on which would be the most suitable without more background detail. You would be wise to make an appointment to see a naturopathic or homoeopathic practitioner.

Is there a treatment for blackheads?
See a qualified beauty therapist, who will remove the blackheads in a responsible and professional manner and advise you on cleansing methods for the skin.

What is the best way to cleanse facial skin?
Definitely not with soap and water. Use a cleansing milk, followed by a cleansing lotion, before putting on day or night cream.

***Acne rosacea* – this appears to be an incurable skin condition. Is there anything that can be done other than giving up certain foods?**
Acne rosacea is very persistent. However, a low stress diet is often helpful (see my book *Stress and Nervous Disorders*). Also, take 15 drops of Echinaforce before meals and ten drops of Petaforce after meals, both twice daily.

What advice would you give to two teenage girls (sisters)

who have a skin problem – 'goose flesh' in layman's terms? The sides of the cheeks, the upper arms, chest and back are all affected. They have had this problem since puberty.
Use Oil of Evening Primrose every day. Also Boldocynara (ten drops after meals, twice daily) and Echinaforce (20 drops before meals, twice daily).

I suffer from a skin complaint that has been diagnosed as a type of condition normally referred to as 'athlete's foot'. After having used ointment for six weeks I still have a skin irritation on the ribs, below the breast area, although there is no itching or pain. What could cause sudden skin eruptions like small burn marks and, more important still, is there a cure? I should tell you that I have never been bothered with skin problems before and I am not aware of any change in my diet that could cause such a condition.
I can understand your concern, but you will be pleased to know that the athlete's foot condition can be treated successfully by dabbing with Molkosan. This is one of Dr Vogel's remedies and is produced in Switzerland from fresh Alpine whey by a natural fermentation process. Molkosan contains all the important minerals found in fresh whey, such as magnesium, potassium and calcium, in concentrated form.

For three years I have had an itchy skin. I have been treated for digestive complaints and liver problems, but nothing has relieved the itching.
I am inclined to believe that the itching is probably caused by a liver condition. Twice a day, take ten drops of Boldocynara in a little water after meals and I would be surprised if the symptoms did not disappear.

SPONDYLOSIS

What can be done for someone with spondylitis or spondylosis?
Both problems can be helped with electro-acupuncture and remedies such as Symphytum, *Harpagophytum*, GS500, or *Arnica 30x*. Both problems are dealt with in more detail in my book *Arthritis, Rheumatism and Psoriasis*.

Four months ago I was diagnosed as having spondylosis in the

lower back. When the problem occurred I had just come off tranquillisers after 21 years. Could there be a connection?
I sincerely doubt if there is a connection. However, with spondylosis a healthy and balanced diet is essential. Also, take selenium and Imperthritica.

What treatment do you recommend for cervical spondylosis?
Acupuncture, laser therapy and Dr Vogel's Detox Box Programme.

STROKES

Is there anything that can be done after a stroke to improve the chances of recovery?
Physiotherapy is essential to try and recover movement in the limbs where it has been lost. Crataegus is a remedy that will be especially useful during this process.

What can you suggest to help people who are recovering from stroke paralysis to regain their muscle power?
Physiotherapy and an all-round supplementary multivitamin preparation will be helpful.

Please tell me about Chelation therapy and tablets to reduce cholesterol.
Chelation is an oral remedy that is made up of vitamins, minerals, trace elements and herbal extracts. I have been able to help many patients over the years with the remedy called FLW.

My mother is 89 years old and over the past few years she has had four mild strokes. For a year now she has suffered from a very dry mouth. She drinks a lot of tap-water.
Perhaps she needs help for some liver disorder. Advise her to drink still mineral water and also to take the two herbal remedies Silymarin and Co-Enzyme Q10. Research has demonstrated that Co-enzyme Q10 (CoQ10), or ubiquinone (from the Latin word meaning 'everywhere'), is essential for the health of all human tissues and organs. It is a 'vitamin-like' substance that is manufactured by the body and is present in the mitochondria of all living cells. The mitochondria are the energy

generators of the cells and the highest proportion of mitochondria are found in these cells that do the most work, notably the liver, muscle tissue and the heart. Researchers are still uncovering the full potential of what leading scientists call the 'biochemical spark' that releases energy from food.

In Japan more than ten million people take CoQ10 daily. Although CoQ10 is found in some foods, the body cannot easily extract it. Moreover, our ability to either absorb or produce it deteriorates as we age. Nutritional deficiencies and genetic or acquired defects can also interfere with the CoQ10 metabolic pathway – a pathway that results in physical energy. People with highly active lifestyles or occupations, including athletes, as well as the elderly, are among those who may choose to take supplementary CoQ10.

My 70-year-old brother has had a number of strokes and is more or less confined to a wheelchair. Over the last few years he has developed an itch, which is apparently systemic (internal). Is there anything you can suggest as a coolant?
For the itch your brother should take Boldocynara (ten drops after meals, twice daily). He would also benefit from CoQ10. For more general advice I would suggest that you read my book *Heart and Blood Circulatory Problems*.

My husband had a stroke more than three years ago and since then he has had trouble with the left side of his body. He also has bad circulation, which he has been told could be due to the fact that he caught chickenpox soon after the stroke. Is there any homoeopathic remedy for this?
Give your husband a combination formula from Dr Vogel called Venosan (15 drops twice daily).

T

THYROID PROBLEMS

What hormone is produced by the thyroid gland?
The thyroid gland produces a hormone called thyroxine. If too much is produced the metabolic rate speeds up and a condition called thyrotoxicosis may occur. If too little of this hormone is produced the metabolism slows down and a condition called myxoedema is the result. To support and balance the thyroid gland take 15 drops of Nasturtium twice daily.

Is there a remedy that can be taken safely for either an over-active or under-active thyroid?
A safe and reliable remedy is Nasturtium. Take ten drops twice daily; if preferred, it can even be mixed through a green salad or used as part of a salad dressing.

Can you please recommend an alternative remedy for an over-active thyroid?
Presumably you are receiving medicine prescribed by your doctor. Alongside this you can safely take a homoeopathic remedy, e.g. *Lycopus virg. 2x, Fucus ves. 3x.* or *Nat. mur. 6x.*

My daughter has a thyroid condition which sometimes causes severe pain in the throat. Any suggestions?
For pain in the throat resulting from thyroid problems your daughter should take the herbal preparation Imperatoria (15 drops twice daily).

What would you suggest for a diminished thyroid function?
One or two Kelpasan tablets daily, taken with a cup of warm water, can often be helpful.

What can I take to wean myself off thyroid medication?

This is not to be advised unless it is done under medical supervision. Please seek the help of a qualified practitioner, who may guide you through this process, while at the same time keeping a close eye on your condition.

I have been told to take Thyroxine for an under-active thyroid. Is there anything I could take that would be more beneficial? I would also be grateful for some advice on my eyes, as they water a great deal because of the thyroid problem.

Thyroxine is a long-term drug which you cannot stop. It will, however, be helpful to take Nasturtium, and for the watery eyes I would recommend Euphrasia officinalis.

I have just been told that my thyroid gland has ceased to function. I would much prefer homoeopathic treatment and would like to hear if you have any suggestions?

Without knowledge of your medical history I am not able to advise you specifically, although you may rest assured that homoeopathy offers help for thyroid problems. I would suggest that you make an appointmnt with a qualified homoeopathic practitioner, who can, together with your GP, work out a suitable programme.

Is it possible to activate an under-active thyroid gland that has been treated with Eltroxin for twenty years?

There is no doubt that help is available, but any treatment should be done under the direct supervision of a qualified homoeopathic practitioner.

How can hypothyroid (an under-active thyroid) be treated naturally?

Diet is very important. A qualified practitioner can give you advice on suitable remedies, and is also likely to recommend three 500 mg capsules of Evening Primrose Oil, to be taken before going to bed.

TONSILITIS

What treatment would you recommend for tonsilitis?
Gargle daily with diluted Molkosan and take *Apis mellificia 3x* and *Lycopodium 6x*. Alternatively, you can gargle with 1.5 per cent hydrogen peroxide.

V

VARICOSE VEINS

What – if any – is the alternative treatment for varicose veins?
In extreme cases the patient should take bed rest and the attention should be concentrated on the circulatory system. Usually, remedies such as *Aesculus hipp.*, Venosan and Urticalcin are prescribed. Dietary instructions are important, e.g. no alcohol, no nicotine, no spices and no salt. Please read my book *Heart and Blood Circulatory Problems*, which devotes a whole chapter to this subject.

Can you advise me if there is a quick remedy to counteract varicose veins?
You must understand that it is impossible to do anything overnight for varicose veins. My book *Heart and Blood Circulatory Problems* contains much advice on this subject and should provide you with a programme that will fit in with your life style.

Do you support the decision to remove varicose veins if they are painful and unsightly? Alternatively, what would you do?
I would always try an alternative first, especially if surgery can be avoided. I have managed to help many people avoid surgery or injections and I would suggest that you read my book *Heart and Blood Circulatory Problems* for more detailed advice.

Last year, on your advice, I took a three-month course of vitamin E for varicose veins, with success. How often does this course need to be repeated?
Preferably twice a year.

I have varicose ulcers which are not healing. Can anything be taken to help?

Unfortunately, varicose ulcers can be a very persistent complaint, and patience is required in their treatment. For internal use take Petaforce, Hyperisan and Urticalcin. Externally, I would suggest poultices made with equal amounts of codliver oil and honey, mixed together and spread on a soft cloth. Lay this on the affected part of the leg, cover with a bandage and leave it in place all night.

VOMITING

My teenage daughter is often sick and vomits several times a week. There appears to be no reason for it.
The best remedy I know is *Nux vomica 3x*. If that does not clear up the condition try *Helianthus tuberosus*.

W

WARTS

Warts can be very persistent. Is there an alternative method to get rid of them?
For external treatment, dab the warts daily with undiluted Molkosan. Internally, take ten drops of *Chelidonium* before meals and ten drops of Petaforce after meals, both twice daily.

My teenage daughter has warts on her fingers and her feet. Is there anything you can recommend?
This condition should be treated as soon as possible because warts have the dreadful habit of spreading. Try *Thuja* and/or *Chelidonium*, both internally and externally, and also dab the affected areas with Molkosan.

WATER QUESTIONS

Are you in favour of adding fluoride to the drinking water?
No, most certainly I am not in favour of this measure. Please read my book *Water – Healer or Poison* and you will learn how I feel about adding fluoride to our drinking water.

What is your opinion or advice on drinking water?
In order to live we require three forms of energy, i.e. food, water and air. The quality of the air we breathe we can do very little about, but we can use our discretion with regard to the quality of both our food and our water. Let us use it wisely!

I live in the Portsmouth area and every day our tap-water tastes of chlorine. It needs to be boiled in order to get rid of

most of the taste. Are any other chemicals used which are not removed by filtering?

Most chemicals that are added to our drinking water are harmless and some of them are sometimes even necessary, e.g chlorides and bromides. Fluoride, however, is not necessary and can be to our detriment. For example, homoeopathic remedies cannot be taken in water that contains fluoride.

Although water filters are good, the cost works out at approximately two pounds per week and as a pensioner I find this too expensive.

Some water filters are more expensive than others. Fortunately, there are now cheaper ways to filter our tap-water.

Is our tap-water today better or worse than it was 50 years ago?

It is, unfortunately, much worse because so many chemicals have been added. Our tap-water should be as pure as possible, because the human body consists mainly of water. There is no point in feeding all this medication involuntarily to the body.

Is water good for panic or anxiety attacks?

Drinking good quality water is always good, although I have never heard of any importance specifically related to panic or anxiety attacks. On average, people drink too little water and if the quality of the water is good one can never drink too much.

My daughter suffers from a water allergy and for the first year she had to be washed with almond oil. Now when she has a shower her skin comes out in blotches and her face burns. Can you help?

In similar cases I have heard that rose water has helped.

I have too much chlorine in my tap-water and get rid of it by filtering. What do you think about that?

Much can be done with a charcoal filter. However, the most harmful substance in the tap-water in some parts of Britain is lead, which, unfortunately, is the most difficult substance to eliminate by filtering.

I suffer from dark circles under my eyes, even though I follow a good diet. I use a charcoal filter and wonder if drinking plenty of water will help?
By installing a charcoal filter you have already taken the most sensible step. Drink plenty of the filtered water and if in doubt ask your doctor to check if there could be anything wrong with the functioning of your kidneys.

Do you really think that we have any say in decisions on measures such as the addition of fluoride to our tap-water? I feel that we are entirely in the hands of so-called 'experts'. Did the World Health Organisation not make strong protestations to the British Government on the fluoride issue?
It appears that public opinion is of little importance in such matters. We must continue to object to unwarranted and unavoidable self-medication.

My son is 11 years old and has never drunk milk in his life. He does drink large quantities of water and suffers badly with catarrh (ever since he was a baby). He has had homoeopathic treatment, i.e. *Phosphorus*. Is the fact that he drinks lots of water a good or a bad thing?
It would be excellent if he drank plenty of *good* water! Please insist that he drinks pure mineral water and he cannot go wrong.

Our tap-water has always come from a well. This water has now been tested and has been approved. Do you think that water drawn from a well has more health benefits than tap-water?
You are lucky, well-water often contains minerals that are advantageous to our health.

Do you have any suggestions on how to remove fluoride from the tap-water for the treatment of arthritis?
It is near enough impossible to filter the water so securely that all fluoride has been removed. Your only option is to use a good-quality mineral water instead.

Can you recommend a good water filter for the Brighton area? Our water tastes strongly of fluoride sometimes.

You may be confusing fluoride with the taste of chlorine, because to my knowledge there is no fluoride in the water in Brighton.

The tap-water in my house tastes awful – like bleach. I have called the Severn Trent Water Authority and they said that additional chlorine in the water was necessary. I now buy bottled water. I have been ill for a long time and now think that the tap-water may be contributing to this. Why must there be so much chlorine in our water?

Being unwell, you are wise to restrict your water intake to bottled water. Alternatively, you could ask to have a sample of your tap-water tested.

The water in my part of the country is very hard and we therefore use a water softener. I would like to hear your views on this. Also, I would like to know if drinking water should be filtered after it has been through the softener?

Usually when a water softener is installed the kitchen tap is isolated because drinking water should not be softened. You will possibly find that this is the case in your home if the system has been installed by a reputable company.

Do you think there will ever be a time when water is delivered to the house in the same way as milk?

This may well happen in the future if our water authorities insist on adding unwanted substances to our tap-water. In that case we will have to invest more in bottled water.

Our water is pumped up from a borehole. We have been told that it is high in nitrates, but nothing else. Is the presence of nitrates in high amounts harmful?

Certainly, nitrates are considered harmful in large quantities. However, certain safe limits have been established and it would be wise to have your water checked to find out whether the level of nitrates exceeds these limits.

I would like to know if it is good or bad to drink boiled water? I drink this in preference to bottled water.

Distilled and boiled water is dead! Water needs life energy in it and therefore I suggest that you either filter your tap-water or drink pure mineral water.

We have a well in the garden and would like to know how to go about getting it in working order to pump it into the house.
A good plumber will be able to help you with this, but first of all I would have the quality of the water tested – before you go to any unproductive expense.

I do not like 'neat' drinking water. Is it as good for you to drink water with lemon and barley water?
Adding lemon and barley water will not do you any harm. The most important thing is to drink plenty of water.

Should fluoride in a public water supply be considered an asset?
I suggest you try and read the most interesting book – *Fluoride – The Freedom Fight*, written by Dr Hans Moolenburgh, and decide for yourself whether this is an asset or a liability.

I have ME and would like to know if my condition makes it more important or less so to use a water purifier?
I would always be in favour of using a water purifier, but never more so than if the person concerned has ME. You should take great care to ensure the quality of the water you drink. If in doubt, use bottled water.

How safe is bottled mineral water and which brands would you recommend?
Most bottled water is safe because it is subject to stringent tests. Personally, I like to use water that has been bottled in glass, in preference to plastic.

Could large intakes of cold tap-water taken on a daily basis be considered as a contributory factor in relation to post-viral debility?
If the water is uncontaminated it is very unlikely that this could have such serious detrimental effects. If you are in doubt about the quality of your water supply you would be wise to get a sample of the water tested.

I don't like tea or coffee and drink a lot of tap-water. Would I benefit by drinking bottled water? Also, do I destroy vitamin C in my drinks by adding hot water?

You are better off drinking tap-water than drinking large quantities of either tea or coffee. In answer to your second question, the vitamin C content is not destroyed by hot water.

Many old pioneers of nature cures had great successes from the therapeutic use of water. Do you use any of these techniques, and if so, how effective are they?
Indeed, I am a great believer in therapeutic water treatments. Many old as well as modern techniques are described in my book *Water – Healer or Poison?*

WEIGHT PROBLEMS

Can you give me some advice on weight loss?
In my book *Realistic Weight Control* you will find a variety of diets to suit individual circumstances and life styles. The general diet given below has been carefully worked out and it has helped many of my patients to lose excess weight.

General diet for weight loss
Daily allowances
Milk – half a pint of fresh or one pint of skimmed, or two cartons of natural yoghurt.
Wholemeal bread – 3 oz (NB not slices).
Meat – 4 oz, *or* 6 oz of fish (smoked fish 4 oz only), *or* 5 oz of chicken.
Fruit – three portions.

Weekly allowances
Butter or margarine – 4 oz, or 8 oz 'Gold'.
Cheese – 8 oz.
Eggs – up to seven (optional).

Exchanges for 1 oz of bread
Potatoes – 3 oz.
Crispbread, crackers or water biscuits, or two plain biscuits.
Breakfast cereal – 1 oz of any variety (not sugar-coated).
Porridge – 1 oz (uncooked weight).
Cooked rice – two dessertspoons.

Variety is the spice of life

Meat: 4 oz daily, cooked in any way, except fried. Beef, corned beef, kidney, lamb, liver, mutton, tongue, tripe, sweetbreads, veal.

Fish: 6 oz daily, cooked in any way, except fried (smoked fish 4 oz only). Crab, cod, haddock, halibut, hake, herrings, kippers, lobster, ling, mackerel, mussels, oysters, pilchards, prawns, salmon, sardines, shrimps, trout, tuna.

Poultry/Game: 5 oz daily, cooked in any way, except fried. Chicken, turkey, rabbit, grouse, pheasant, venison.

Eggs: One medium egg daily (optional) cooked in any way, except fried.

Cheese: 1 oz daily (except cottage cheese). Caerphilly, Camembert, Cheddar, Cheshire, cottage (4 oz), Danish Blue, Edam, Gruyère, Leicester, Parmesan, Roquefort, Stilton, Wensleydale, smoked Austrian.

Vegetables: (Unlimited) Artichokes, asparagus, aubergines, bean sprouts, beetroot, broccoli, cabbage (any type), cauliflower, celery, carrots, cress, cucumber, courgettes, chicory, leeks, lettuce, marrow, mushrooms, onions, peppers, pimentos, parsnip, pickles, parsley, French and runner beans, radishes, swede, spring onions, spinach, tomatoes.

(In moderation) Avocado, baked beans (3–5 oz), beans (broad, butter, haricot), chickpeas, peas, sweetcorn.

Fruit: These portions daily:

Apple	– 1 average	Peach	– 1 average
Apricots	– 2 fresh	Pear	– 1 average
Bananas	– 1 small	Pineapple	– 1 slice fresh
Blackberries	– 4 oz	Plums	– 2 fresh
Cooking apple	– 1 large	Pomegranate	– 1 small
Cherries	– 4 oz	Prunes	– 6 stewed
Dates	– 1 oz	Raisins	– 1 oz
Damsons	– 10	Raspberries	– 5 oz
Gooseberries	– 10	Rhubarb	– 5 oz
Grapefruit	– half	Strawberries	– 5 oz
Grapes	– 3 oz	Sultanas	– 1 oz
Melon	– 1 average slice	Tangerines, etc.	– 2
Orange	– 1 average	Unsweetened juice	– 4 fl oz

Drinks: Tea (including Russian tea), herb tea, coffee, Bovril, Oxo, Marmite, soda water, lemon juice, tomato juice, water, Energen 1-Cal, slimline drinks, low-calorie tonic.

Seasonings: Salt, pepper, vinegar, mustard, lemon juice, herbs, spices, Worcester sauce.

Points to note:
1. Your daily allowance must be consumed within a period of 24 hours.
2. Eat your weekly allowance within one week.
3. You may eat as often as you like within your allowance.
4. However, you must not eat fewer than three meals a day.

I must lose weight because I have diverticulitis, pain right through the back and weakness in the stomach. What would you advise?
With any health problems one should take special care with the diet. You may like to read my book *Stomach and Bowel Problems* which gives much dietary detail, or I would suggest that you consult a dietician for advice specific to your circumstances.

I have been treated for irritable bowel syndrome for many years with Colofac and Fybogel and a high-fibre diet – mainly bran-based. About ten months ago I changed from bran to Linoforce with some improvement, but feel unhappy and probably over-treated with my present condition. I am also overweight. I consider I have a good, balanced diet, though no doubt I ought to eat more fruit and vegetables. I have a demanding job which places some limitations on my eating habits. What help could alternative treatment offer? Also, please advise on some satisfying alternatives to drinking tea? (I do not drink coffee or alcohol.)
With respect to your question on diet, follow the diet given above. As to your second question, Bambu is a coffee substitute, which can also be considered as an alternative to tea. You could also try some herbal teas, e.g. peppermint, rose hip or camomile.

Does a craving for certain foods, e.g. wheat or dairy products suggest an allergy to those foods?

It is often the case that the foods one eats most are those one is allergic to. If in doubt, check this with your practitioner.

Do you know of a natural appetite depressant?

Fucus Ves. or Vogel's Slimming Formula can both be used for this purpose. However, remember that it is the change in eating habits that is important when trying to lose weight and that is not obtained by depressing one's appetitite. Any such appetite-depressant should only be used short-term.

How should one approach losing weight?

Always positively! The only way to successfully lose weight is with a positive attitude. Keep to the diet, but realise that the mental approach is equally important.

How does slimming by acupuncture work? Does it alter the metabolism?

Acupuncture helps to speed up the metabolism and is therefore a very effective aid to losing weight.

Is it possible that the lack of a certain vitamin causes compulsive over-eating?

You are quite right, because a particular deficiency can often be the cause of a specific compulsion or over-indulgence. This factor is dealt with in my book *Realistic Weight Control*.

My daughter is 36 years old and appears to have a very slow metabolism. She has been told to take kelp. Have you heard of these tablets and what do you think? My daughter also has a very nervous disposition.

In cases of a slow metabolism kelp often works. Unless there are thyroid problems one can take up to four tablets of Kelpasan a day – to be taken first thing in the morning with a cup of warm water.

Apart from weight control, what would your advice be for hypertension?

Be careful with salt intake. Follow a low-stress diet and possibly take Arterioforce (one capsule three times a day).

What can I do to gain weight?

Eat plenty of nuts, potatoes, bananas, soya, etc. Take 15 drops of Centaurium twice daily.

Please suggest an appetite-stimulant for a frail 80-year-old lady.
Take 15 drops of *Centaurium* in half a cup of water and one teaspoon of Vitaforce, both twice daily.

I only take one meal a day – no breakfast and no evening meal. Since the death of my husband I have lost two stones and still continue to lose weight. I am now worried that I am losing too much weight, but I have no appetite. What can I do about it?
Start by taking some *Ignatia 3x*, which will help you to overcome the grief of your husband's death. Then take, twice daily, 15 drops of *Centaurium*, some wheatgerm capsules and Vitaforce.

WORMS

What can be done about a long-term problem with worms? Would your advice also be applicable to children?
Always eat plenty of onions, leeks and garlic. Remember that all papaya products are also good under these circumstances. Therefore take one or two tablets of Papayasan twice daily. This treatment is also suitable for children.

MISCELLANEOUS

This section features somes of the wide-ranging questions I have been asked at public lectures over the years. The diversity of the topics covered made it difficult to catalogue them in any of the more specific sections contained in this book, and therefore I have decided to include this 'Miscellaneous' section where the reader can browse. I have also included here a number of questions which are fairly similar, and yet different, to some of the questions dealt with in the specific sections. Yet again, I must point out that, although I will always attempt to answer people to the best of my knowledge, without full details of the questioner's medical background the help I can give is limited to more general recommendations. For this reason I would always suggest that the reader, whenever possible, consult a doctor or alternative practitioner for individual advice.

After work I like to stop off with my friends for a drink. How much can I drink and still be safe to drive home?
Even the smallest quantity of alcohol will affect your ability to drive. Moreover, alcohol is never safe because it is addictive. Be careful!

The doctor wants me to have a smear test. Do I have cancer?
The smear test is not a cancer test. This test is specifically designed to detect any pre-cancerous conditions.

How much help is the visualisation therapy for physical conditions?
A positive approach is always important, whether the person's complaints are physical or psychological. A healthy mind – a healthy body! Always be positive, irrespective of how serious the physical condition may be. Visualise a healthy body and never forget the counterbalance of positive and negative thinking.

What is your advice for Pfeiffer's disease?

This illness first was diagnosed around the turn of the century by a German doctor whose name was given to the disease. It is more commonly known as glandular fever. The main symptoms are epidemic tiredness, fever and glandular swelling, often together with anaemia. It primarily affects the younger generation and is thought to be caused by a virus. Its treatment includes taking plenty of rest and drinking plenty of fruit juices and herbal teas – Jan de Vries' Herbal Tea is especially suitable. Recommended remedies for Pfeiffer's disease are Echinaforce, *Spongia* and Imuno-Strength.

I am 30 years of age and have a rare bone disease – Engelman's disease – which I have had all my life. In the past I have tried homoeopathic remedies (various tissue salts) without benefit. At present I am taking prescribed painkillers and will have to go back on steroids. Can you suggest an alternative?

Try taking five Urticalcin tablets and one ArMax capsule twice daily.

Can you suggest any treatment for sarcoidosis?

Sarcoidosis is a relatively obscure disease, symptomised by granular growths in the organs, joints, bones and lymph glands. Its causes are unknown, although it is thought that genetic factors are involved. A homoeopathic practitioner may be able to prescribe for some of the specific symptoms after examining you.

What is Reiter's syndrome? Is it common and what do you suggest as a remedy?

Reiter's syndrome is not a common disease, but can be a great nuisance. It is a peripheral arthritis in association with urethritis. Sometimes the remedy GS500 helps and this should be taken in combination with Petaforce capsules.

Please tell me the causes of a 'runny' nose and what treatment you would suggest.

It is possible that this is caused by an allergy, but that cannot be substantiated without further tests. I would recommend that you take, three times daily, ten drops of Formula SNS, together with some Urticalcin tablets.

What can I do about continuous problems of infected mucus entering the mouth from the sinuses?
Take one tablet of SinuCheck three times a day.

What do you recommend for bad breath caused by nasal catarrh?
Antibiotics only give a short-term relief. Take 15 drops of Echinaforce before meals twice daily and three garlic capsules before going to bed.

I have read that raspberry leaf tea is good for lowering the blood pressure. Mine came down from 190/90 to 130/70. Is there any harm in taking it too often or long-term?
It cannot do any harm and many people find it quite a pleasant drink.

What do you recommend for the treatment of Hodgkin's disease?
Read the description of this condition and the advice on general treatment methods in my book *Cancer and Leukaemia*.

Please could you recommend a homoeopathic or naturopathic pain reliever for sinus-type headaches?
Take two tablets of Petaforce twice daily before meals.

What dietary supplement can one take to ensure strength and vitality?
Twice a day, take one tablet of Health Insurance Plus – a most sensible vitamin and mineral supplement.

What do you recommend for hot flushes?
Take 15 drops of *Menosan* in a little water twice daily.

Can catarrh aggravated by a nasal polyp be helped without resorting to surgery to remove the polyp?
Try taking 15 drops of *Marum verum* for a minimum of three months. If this is not effective you still have the option of undergoing surgery.

How do you break a child's 'bad' eating habits without creating too much unpleasantness?
There is no easy answer to this question, but it is certainly a worthwhile

exercise. Do it in a very relaxed way and gradually. Only healthy foods are required by the body, but this is difficult to explain to a child.

Is there anything I can take to regulate my menstrual cycle?

Take PMS Formula and also read my book *Menstrual and Pre-Menstrual Tension*.

Can anything be done to help people with Huntington's chorea?

This is a difficult condition to treat, but I have seen some encouraging results in patients treated with the Fresh Cell Therapy from Professor Niehans.

I have a very low energy level and suffer from depression. Can you suggest a remedy?

Try taking two tablets of Ginsavita and two tablets of Imuno-Strength, both twice daily.

Is there such a thing as 'growing pains'? This question is in specific relation to children aged 7–14 who complain of aches and pains in the joints.

Growing pains can be caused by various conditions, either hormonal, congenital or others. A homoeopathic practitioner will probably prescribe a constitutional remedy, but it is always good to supplement the children's diets with zinc.

I get a clicking noise in the right side of my head. Is it an ear problem or is it arthritis?

It could be either – without further investigation or examination details I cannot advise you. Consult a qualified osteopath or chiropractor for the correct diagnosis and treatment advice.

I have been told that I have slight osteoporosis. Can I prevent this getting worse?

Take five Urticalcin tablets twice daily.

Can *Ginkgo biloba* be given to a very elderly person?

Very much so; elderly people will benefit greatly from taking this food supplement.

What do you think of *Agnus castus* – the herb used in the treatment for pre-menstrual syndrome?
Indeed, this is a most effective herb for helping people who suffer from pre-menstrual tension.

I am in my mid sixties. Two years ago I broke my femur. Should I take calcium?
You will find that taking five Urticalcin tablets twice daily will be very helpful.

Should *Echinacea* be taken for only short periods of time? Is its continuous use dangerous in any way?
There is no danger if the guidelines for the recommended dosage are followed.

Why am I craving chocolate and what can I do about it?
Remember that sugar and chocolate are just as addictive as nicotine and alcohol. If you are worried you may decide to try acupuncture to stop this addiction.

How can I cope with tiredness and pre-menstrual tension?
Take PMS Formula and Optivite. For more detailed advice read my book *Menstrual and Pre-Menstrual Tension*.

I have Parkinson's disease and would like to know what I can do about the side-effects of Sinumet?
The side-effects of Sinumet can be helped by taking ten drops of Boldocynara twice daily after meals.

Do you think some of the 'torment' suffered by a severely mentally handicapped child could be caused by the malalignment of the spine and, if so, could manipulation (or other treatment) bring relief?
Cranial osteopathy could be extremely helpful in such cases.

What can I do for a recurring tooth abcess?
At the first signs of discomfort take *Belladonna 30*.

What do you think are the barriers against natural remedies being integrated into the present medical system? How do

you think these barriers can be overcome?
By perseverance and change in the economic and political approach.

I am 60 years old and have been a walker all my life. I am on a low-fat diet and under treatment for high blood pressure and high cholesterol. Now arthritis has appeared, in spite of diuretic tablets. I am almost a vegetarian and would like to know if I should take fish-oil tablets?
Fish-oil tablets will be helpful for both your arthritic condition and your blood pressure.

I get easily confused and am inclined to forget where I leave my keys, etc. Can I take tablets to improve my memory? I am in my sixties, live alone and feel lonely.
Read my book *Heart and Blood Circulatory Problems* and take Imuno-Strength as a general food supplement.

What do you suggest for hay fever and dry skin problems?
These problems could well be interlinked and therefore both should be treated. For the hay fever take Pollinosan and for the skin I would recommend Oil of Evening Primrose capsules.

What do you think about taking Chinese herbs to build up one's immune system, as well as following a natural diet?
Opting to follow a natural diet is always a sensible decision. There are quite a number of Chinese herbs available now in the West, although some are for general purposes, while others have a more specific application. Traditional Chinese practitioners, however, possess a wealth of knowledge which only now are we slowly learning about and coming to accept in the West.

Do you believe that orthodox and alternative medicine complement each other and that their practitioners can work together successfully?
Most definitely, because it is, or should be, every practitioner's aim to reduce human suffering.

I have a brother who lives in England and another who lives in Ireland. I spoke to them recently and both seem to be

experiencing pain and problems from intermittent claudication. What treatment would you advise?

Please advise your brothers to read my book *Heart and Blood Circulatory Problems* for general suggestions. For intermittent claudication I would not hesitate to prescribe Vasolastine injections, which I have used very successfully for many years. *Ginkgo biloba* and Chelation Therapy are also excellent for this condition.

Where can we obtain a copy of the book *The Nature Doctor?*

Bioforce UK will be able to send you a copy and the address can be found in this book under the section 'Useful addresses'.

I have pains in hands, shoulders and back. I do not know why and would like to know what to do.

Please read my book *Neck and Back Problems* for general dietary and remedial advice.

Do ionisers work?

You should always follow the manufacturer's instructions. Most of the feedback from people who have invested in an ioniser has been very positive.

Since my mother's friend stopped smoking she has experienced many side-effects. She has not been well since she stopped and as we are trying to get my mother to stop, could you please explain why this friend should have reacted so unfavourably?

The chemical dependency on nicotine can indeed have side-effects and therefore I always advise people who are giving up smoking to initially use a homoeopathic tobacco substitute called *Tabacum D4*.

Very soon I will have to stay over in hospital for the extraction of two impacted wisdom teeth. Apart from *Arnica* tablets, can you recommend anything to aid the healing afterwards?

Also take 15 drops of Echinaforce twice daily.

How is ALS (amyothrophic lateral sclerosis) related to food or nutrition? How would you treat it?

In cases of ALS it is very possible that there is a lack of amino acids in the daily diet. This would be the area I would investigate first.

I have suffered from *Hyperemesis gravitas* and post-natal depression with both of my children. There appear to be two approaches to this: psychosomatic or hormonal. Can you advise me please?
Take zinc and *Valeriana* drops before and after the birth. Also take Oil of Evening Primrose capsules afterwards.

How would you deal with a persistent sore throat?
Take one tablet of *Hepar sulph. 3x* three times a day.

What symptoms might one expect with a calcium deficiency?
In the condition of the hair and nails, deterioration, tiredness and anaemia are often experienced.

I am an air hostess. Could you please advise me on how to cope with flight fatigue, changes in air pressure, breathing re-cycled air and negative energy flow?
Twice a day take 15 drops of *Ginkgo biloba*. If a special boost is needed, take two tablets of Ginsavita – also twice daily.

What is the treatment for colitis in dogs?
Add, twice daily, five drops of Tormentavena to your pet's drinking water.

Could you please give a brief outline of what H_2O_2 is?
H_2O_2 is hydrogen peroxide. This substance should be used under medical supervision only.

What is your opinion of ginseng?
Ginseng is very good for increasing one's level of activity. However, I must emphasise that patients with heart conditions are not advised to use this remedy.

My mother is 88 years of age and keeps getting chest infections. How can they be prevented and what treatment can she have other than antibiotics, which do not agree with her?

Give elderly people 15 drops of Echinaforce and half a teaspoon of Drosinula syrup in half a cup of hot water, both twice daily.

What can one take for migraine headaches?
Twice daily, take 15 drops of *Loranthus*. Read the section on 'Migraines' in this book.

My husband has pain and numbness just above the knee. He is taking Brufen, but we would like to know if this complaint could be due to stress?
Because of the lack of detail I cannot comment on the possible stress factor. I would suggest that before going to bed he places a cabbage leaf over the affected area and binds this into place with a soft bandage. He should keep this on overnight and repeat the procedure every alternate night.

Please explain how to use the thumbs, which are neutral, for self-healing purposes.
You will find a complete explanation, together with many sample exercises, in my book *Body Energy*.

I wear soft contact lenses and want to continue wearing them for as long as possible. Yet I am rather worried about the chemical disinfectant solution I have to use. Can you advise on anything I can do to counteract any adverse effects the lenses may have?
There is a Swiss eye lotion called Oculosan which is excellent for cleaning the eyes. This should be used approximately three times per week.

If one has been advised to stop drinking tea or coffee, what substitutes can be used?
Tea can easily be replaced by a variety of herbal teas, and there is an excellent coffee substitute called Bambu.

What can be done to alleviate a fear of going out alone?
Talk it over with family and friends and I am confident that you will find them very supportive. Please read my book *Stress and Nervous Disorders* and take the remedy Aconite.

What would you recommend for my little girl's nosebleeds? She is eight years old.
Give her five drops of *Hamamelis virg.* (witch hazel) twice daily.

Can you tell us the effects of drinking coffee and what would happen if the habit was discontinued?
Caffeine can cause a number of problems and I would recommend that you read about this in my book *Nature's Gift of Food*. Going without coffee may cause a few headaches initially.

Is there such a thing as a 'sick office syndrome'? If there is, how can it be measured and how can it be corrected?
Sometimes neon strip lights may have a detrimental effect on the people working under such conditions, as can air-conditioning and recycled air. However, it could easily be influenced by the visual display screens of computers and word processors. The effects of such factors are difficult to measure. If you have no choice but to work under these conditions, try to compensate by taking plenty of exercise and fresh air.

Is it true that people with a tendency towards epilepsy should not take Evening Primrose Oil?
Correct. I always advise patients with migraine or epilepsy not to take Evening Primrose Oil.

What would you recommend for a small baby who at 14 weeks of age has already had two spells in hospital on antibiotics. The first time it was with a chest infection and the second time with a stomach infection, although at the hospital no reason for the infection could be found. This baby is bottle-fed, but he has also had a skin rash diagnosed as thrush.
Give the baby five drops of Echinaforce twice daily. This will help to fight off infections.

Can benign cysts be removed without surgery?
Sometimes this is possible and I would suggest that you take ten drops of Petaforce twice daily after meals.

For two years – ever since my husband's death – I have been troubled with a dry cough. It comes suddenly and really hurts.
Take 15 drops of Echinaforce twice daily, before meals and also 15 drops of Usneasan twice daily after meals.

Is there any help for cystic fibrosis?
Cystic fibrosis is a difficult condition, but a good homoeopath should be able to help you and ease the symptoms.

My son has had a chronic problem with boils for years. What can he do?
Advise your son to take *Merc. solub. C5x* and also, twice daily, ten drops of Petaforce.

I have recently been to hospital for breast surgery, but my wound does not seem to be healing very well. Is there a vitamin that could help?
Take three 500 mg capsules of Oil of Evening Primrose at night and twice a day take ten drops of Petasan.

Is there a herbal remedy for moles? I know that there is one for warts and veruccas, but I understand that moles are different.
For moles the general recommendation is to take 15 drops of *Chelidonium* twice daily.

How would you go about treating irregular menstruation?
Take ten drops of PMS Formula twice daily and two Optivite tablets per day.

I am female and in my mid-forties. Should I start taking a calcium supplement?
This is not a bad idea as long as it is a calcium preparation that can be readily absorbed by the body. The calcium content of our diet is depleted by food processing and refining techniques and anyone who eats little or no dairy produce should take special care to ensure an adequate intake of calcium. Calcium is the most abundant mineral in the body, 99 per cent of which is used for the bones and teeth. The calcium in our bones is not static, but moves continuously between the blood and the bones. Calcium is also found inside the body cells, where it is needed for the transmission of nerve impulses to the muscles and heart. It is also needed for maintaining the tone and elasticity of our muscles, including the heart, and it is a factor in blood clotting. Calcium is further associated with the use of amino acids and with hormone production. Its function is closely linked with magnesium.

My husband has to get up four or five times a night to go to the bathroom. His doctor has given him a good examination for prostate trouble and everything is all right. Can you recommend anything?

Although the prostate is all right, he will no doubt benefit from Prostabrit, a relatively new remedy in the UK, but most beneficial for complaints such as your husband's.

My 15-year-old niece has been diagnosed as suffering from inflammatory bowel disease. What treatment would you recommend?

Dietary instructions can be found in my book *Stomach and Bowel Disorders*. Applicable remedies are peppermint capsules and Tormentavena (ten drops, twice daily after meals).

When someone has had acupuncture treatment to help her give up smoking and has managed to stop for a few weeks, then has a desire to start again, can she have extra treatment later?

Usually one treatment session is enough, but if the person concerned feels happier with an extra session, there is no reason why that should not take place.

What would you give to a person with endometriosis?

Take Oil of Evening Primrose capsules and the homoeopathic remedy *Ovarium*.

What treatment would you recommend for cold sores?

Twice a day, take 15 drops of Echinaforce before meals.

How do you treat coughing in young children? It seems to just come and go. There is no pattern and sometimes it is wet and other times dry.

Give the child ten drops of Echinaforce twice daily.

What is best for someone who is lacking in iron?

One of the best iron supplements is Iron Plus from Nature's Best.

I have spina bifida and currently take Equiset and Minoforce together with Evening Primrose and garlic. However, what is

bothering me lately is the arthritis in my knees. It is not even the pain so much, but the fact that my legs keep jumping in bed at night from the knee and I cannot control them. This keeps me awake at night.

You will be very much helped by the remedy named ArMax from Enzymatic Therapy, as well as Folic Acid.

Is it possible for a person to suffer from hypoglycaemia only when in a stress situation?

Stress is responsible for many problems and is thought to affect the endocrine system. Therefore stress can indeed cause hypoglycaemia.

What treatment do you suggest for glandular fever, which affects so many teenagers nowadays?

Echinaforce and Urticalcin are both helpful for glandular fever.

My 19-year-old daughter suffers with bad periods, accompanied by sickness, pain and diarrhoea. She has been taking Evening Primrose Oil three times a day. Is this good or have you any other suggestions?

Perhaps your daughter would benefit from reading my book *Menstrual and Pre-Menstrual Tension*. But certainly, taking Oil of Evening Primrose is always beneficial.

How can *Echinacea* be taken? To boost the immune system can it be taken in a small dose over a long time or just for a short period?

Recent tests have proved that there is no harm in taking *Echinacea* over a long-term period.

Will a person taking homoeopathic remedies for a specific complaint sometimes get worse before any improvement shows?

This occurrence is quite usual with homoeopathic medication and is known as the 'healing crisis'. However, the initial poor reaction is encouraging because it indicates that the medicine is effective and will eventually lead to improvement or a cure.

Should one have amalgam (mercury) dental fillings removed?

Is it also possible to keep the fillings and resort to routine body-cleansing to maintain health?
It is better to have the fillings replaced. It is also advisable to take high dosages of Echinaforce during and after the dental treatment.

In your view can Evening Primrose Oil – without any other medication – help for endometriosis, even the bowel version?
Whether no other medication is required depends on the severity of the disease, but you may rest assured that Evening Primrose Oil will always be helpful.

Do you have any suggestions for helping a person with endometriosis?
There are various approaches and I would strongly advise you to consult a qualified practitioner for help.

Can you recommend anything to speed up the healing process and also help with oedema following a troublesome hysterectomy some 12 months ago?
Take three capsules of Oil of Evening Primrose every night before going to bed.

Do you know what causes vitiligo and is there any treatment to stop it spreading?
Sometimes it is a topical influence, but often it is caused by a vitamin or mineral deficiency. A well-balanced vitamin and mineral supplement may therefore be of considerable help.

What practical methods can we use to influence our Government towards recognition of holistic medicine?
The best way may be to approach your own MP and seek support in your own constituency.

How do you personally, as an alternative practitioner, feel about the contraceptive pill?
As an alternative practitioner I must admit that I would not prescribe this method of birth control for my own wife. Whether a woman takes it or not must remain the free choice we are fortunate to have in this country, but I usually point out that there are other methods that are less intrusive on our health.

With so many of our vegetables and fruit being subjected to chemical sprays, how is it possible to live 'naturally' and how can we detoxify our bodies?

We can aim to eat organically grown food wherever possible. If this proves difficult to obtain, we can use Nature's Best's Detoxifying Formula or Dr Vogel's Detox Box Programme.

What can be done about herpes on the face?

For external use I strongly recommend the 7 Herb Cream, while for internal use I would suggest taking one Viraplex capsule together with 20 drops of Echinaforce, twice daily.

What does it mean when the instructions accompanying homoeopathic remedies state 'not suitable for babies'? At what age would it be safe to give a child homoeopathic medicine?

Young children and babies can only take a third of the dosage of an adult. Children from six to 12 years can be given half the adult dosage and children from 12 onwards can take the adult dosage.

My grandson is three years old and sometimes gets frightful attacks of croup. What can be done?

If the croup attack is severe you must always call the doctor without delay. It is of great help to immediately give him Aconite 30x and if the attack persists also give him *Merc. solub. 5x* or *Spongia 6x*.

May I have your suggestions on how to help someone cope with grief?

Make sure that person knows that you are there for him or her to talk about that grief. There is no more worthwhile medicine for a grief-stricken or lonely person than knowing that someone is sympathetic to one's problem. For more specific advice on remedies I would suggest that you refer to my book *Stress and Nervous Disorders*.

Can you recommend any remedies for mouth ulcers?

Be careful with your sugar intake and take twice daily half a teaspoon of Molkosan in half a cup of water.

What about someone who has never been breastfed and now has many deficiency problems, as well as a lactose intolerance?
Take four Urticalcin tablets twice daily.

I am an artist and paint for long periods with oil paints. Could this cause problems? Can I read up on this?
My book *Viruses, Allergies and the Immune System* deals with problems or questions such as yours. Remember that it is good to detoxify the body as often as possible. Take plenty of fresh air and use Nature's Best's Detoxification Formula.

I recently read in an article that living near high-voltage electricity cables could cause health problems and that even vegetables or crops grown in fields in close proximity to these cables would be affected. Also, in another article it was stated that living near mushroom-growing units could cause health problems. What is your opinion?
In my book *Body Energy* I have written extensively on this subject. The health risks, especially of the former case you refer to, posed by such factors are becoming more widely acknowledged now. Geopathic stress has become a real problem.

From time to time I develop lumps on my arms and legs. They are not sore unless touched and usually last no longer than 48 hours. They tend to look inflamed before they subside and finally disappear. My doctor has been unable to discover the cause of these lumps and I would like to hear if you have any suggestions?
Without a medical examination I have not much to go by, but I can assure you that the homoeopathic remedy *Merc. solub.* 5x is always beneficial. Also take Petaforce (ten drops twice daily).

I have heard you talk about vitamin C and would greatly appreciate being able to read about it because I have not been able to remember all the information you gave.
Vitamin C is a unique nutrient, known to be involved either directly, or as a link somewhere in the chain, in at least 300 biochemical pathways in the body. It is an essential water-soluble vitamin that cannot be stored in

the body and much of the vitamin content in a meal will be excreted within four hours. Unlike most animals, human beings can no longer synthesise it. We have to obtain it every day from our food.

Vitamin C, being one of the fragile water-soluble nutrients, is highly unstable and easily destroyed by heat and light, and it is not always possible to be sure how much is being taken in the diet. Our daily requirement of vitamin C is higher than for any other water-soluble vitamin. Much of the vitamin C content of our food is lost through the processes of storing, peeling, freezing and cooking. Nature's Best offers an extensive range of vitamin C supplements for people who wish to safeguard their intake, since our daily intake fluctuates greatly and it is held to be the single most important nutrient.

As a nutrient vitamin C is needed for:

- the production of collagen, a tough, fibrous protein which is an integral part of the skin, tendons, bones, gums, teeth and blood vessels;

- the synthesis of brain and nerve messengers;

- as a protective anti-oxidant throughout the body via its role as a free radical scavenger;

- maintaining the immune system;

- maintaining healthy bones, teeth and gums;

- helping to maintain normal blood fat and cholesterol levels;

- efficient body repair and maintenance;

- fat metabolism.

The most common and richest food sources of this vitamin include the citrus fruits, blackcurrants, acerola cherries, parsley and green vegetables. The categories of people who may choose to supplement their dietary intake are:

- people who consume diets devoid of fresh fruit and vegetables or have particular nutritional requirements, such as the elderly, and those who are dependent on institutional catering;

- smokers and those who drink alcohol;

- those with demanding life styles or occupations and whose diets are inadequate;

- those wishing to maintain normal blood fats and cholesterol.

- people who use aspirin, or take prescribed drugs such as antibiotics or the contraceptive pill;

- athletes and those whose occupation involves vigorous physical activity;

- anyone convalescing from surgical or accidental wounds.

Vitamin C also plays a role in the effective utilisation and metabolism of other nutrients. Folic acid is converted to its biochemically active form with the help of vitamin C, whilst iron will not be efficiently absorbed by the body unless there is sufficient vitamin C present. Zinc together with vitamin C work to maintain the immune system. Water-soluble vitamin C also acts as a roaming scavenger complementing the effects of vitamins E and A as the main anti-oxidants within the cells. The B-complex vitamins and vitamin C are used more rapidly when the body is subjected to demanding situations.

Unfortunately, I suffer terribly with a very sore bottom lip. The symptoms are a sensation of tingling and burning and then it swells up and the skin breaks. It must be an allergy and I suffer especially in the summer. Can you offer any advice?

You may be right in that it is caused by an allergy, but you should have it treated. If your doctor cannot help you try taking ten drops of Petaforce twice daily before meals and ten drops of Echinaforce twice daily after meals.

Someone told me that we should not wear shoes with rubber soles. Is that true?

In general, shoes with leather soles are to be preferred, because rubber soles are thought to reduce assimilation.

I suffer from osteoarthritis in the spine and hips, but my main problem is dragging pains down both thighs and also numbness in my left foot and toes. Is it possible that the

sciatic nerve is trapped? I have been examined by a vascular specialist for my circulation and been given the all-clear.

I would advise that you take 15 drops of Imperthritica together with two ArMax tablets, both twice daily, and am confident that you will soon feel some improvement.

During the last five years I have been subject to epileptic fits, due to a slight stroke which has left a scar on the brain. I am also going through the change of life and have an under-active thyroid. I would like to know if the scar will ever heal and if I can expect the fits to stop? Does the change of life and the thyroid condition have any bearing on the fits?

It is probable that the thyroid condition does have some impact on the fits. Try taking twice daily 15 drops of *Loranthus* twice a day before meals in half a cup of water.

What are your thoughts on reflexology?

Reflexology is a most useful and effective treatment method and you can read more about this therapy in my book *Body Energy*.

I frequently suffer from depression and travel sickness and would like to know if there is an alternative medicine for travel sickness, i.e. different from the usual chemical pills?

Take ten drops of *Nux vomica D4* twice daily.

What would you advise for recurring laryngitis?

Take 20 drops of Echinaforce twice daily.

I am a veterinary nurse and would like to hear your views on the use of homoeopathic medicine for animals. Where can I obtain information on this?

There is much evidence on how well animals respond to homoeopathic remedies and treatment. I have treated a number of horses and the results have been remarkable. If you are looking for more information on this subject I would suggest that you contact one of the homoeopathic hospitals, where they will be able to advise you.

I would like to know what you would suggest for motion vertigo?

Take 15 drops of *Ginkgo biloba* twice daily.

I can only think that I have had some kind of virus for the last two years. I have had various blood tests, but no-one is able to identify this virus. I am, however, losing my hair. Is there anything I can take?

The information I have is too limited to make a sensible suggestion. In order to do so, I would have to examine you. As you appear to be convinced that you have been struck by a virus, I can only suggest that you read my book *Viruses, Allergies and the Immune System*.

Can you please give me some advice on how to treat a baker's cyst?

Rub the cyst with castor oil every night and every other night wrap a cabbage leaf over it.

I have had great success using single remedies. Do you advocate using combination remedies rather than single remedies?

I often start with single remedies and may progress to combination remedies. You should understand, however, that this is largely dependent upon the circumstances and the patient's condition.

What would help for adhesions?

Take three 500 mg capsules of Oil of Evening Primrose before bedtime.

Can earth energy be harmful and is it possible that electric power cables can influence the mains water?

In my book *Body Energy* you will be able to read my views on this subject.

In your book *Arthritis, Rheumatism and Psoriasis* I read that you do not recommend concrete flooring for arthritic people. What is the best type of flooring?

The best material for flooring for anyone – not only for arthritis sufferers – is wood. Wood is a natural product and is conductive. Concrete and cement floors cut the energy fields, which should be allowed to complete a circle.

I have heard that you recommend diets for people suffering from diabetes, MS and many more illnesses. I would therefore like to know if you also have any dietary advice for

cancer patients, like me? I have lost a lot of weight and would like to hear your advice on how to put some of it back on.
Such advice can be found in my book *Cancer and Leukaemia*.

Is there a naturopathic or homoeopathic drink to clear or flush all toxins out of the body system? I have heard that drinking only water for a whole day may act as a purifier for the body.
Dr Vogel's Detox Box Programme has been specifically designed for this purpose.

I suffer greatly from sinus problems and recently I have had five nose haemorrhages in two weeks, lasting for two hours each. Have you any suggestions?
Twice a day take ten drops of Formula SNS together with two SinuCheck tablets.

Some two or three years ago I lost my voice and now I can only speak in a whisper. I have attended speech therapy, but my voice has not come back and I am getting very upset about this. Have you any suggestions on how to improve on the present situation?
This is often caused by a deficiency in iron, and it is also worth remembering that such a condition can often be helped by acupuncture treatment.

I have palpitations and also chronic constipation. Is there anything that can help with this?
The palpitations may disappear if the constipation is treated. To avoid constipation chew half a teaspoon of Linoforce granules twice daily.

Is there a cure for seeing stars in front of your eyes? I have been taking some medication for blood pressure recently, but I am still seeing stars.
If your blood pressure has been checked and regulated I would advise that you take 15 drops of Venosan twice daily.

I have been diagnosed as suffering from a condition called SLE and recently I have taken three *grand mal* fits. After the first I was told that this was an isolated incident and this would not happen again. Subsequently I have had two more attacks. I would like to know if I have developed epilepsy or do I still have SLE?

SLE (sytemic lupus erythemathosis) is an auto-immune problem. The epilepsy is a neurological one. Therefore it is not likely that the epilepsy is caused by the lupus problem. Either condition can be treated by alternative remedies in conjunction with orthodox treatment.

What do you recommend for recurrent vaginal thrush?

For a period of time you should limit your intake of fresh fruit and vegetables. Also, take 15 drops of Nephrosolid twice daily.

What can be done about intestinal problems?

These should be investigated by a qualified practitioner, after which you may be advised to take ten drops of Tormentavena twice daily.

What is the alternative approach to chronic rhinitis?

A very good remedy for this condition is Formula SNS: ten drops taken twice daily.

Is it bad to drink espresso coffee each morning?

Coffee is an addictive substance, although a limited intake cannot do much harm unless one is allergic to it. In most cases I would suggest drinking no coffee at all.

My problem is ulcerations on the legs which can take up to a year to heal. They seem to turn septic for no reason at all. I am taking water tablets and blood pressure tablets. Is there anything I can take to prevent the ulcerations?

Prevention is better than cure and therefore I would suggest that you take 2g of vitamin C every day. Also take ten drops of Petaforce and two Imuno-Strength tablets twice daily.

I have heard that *Thuja* tablets should be taken for warts and this I have done, but I now suffer from diarrhoea as a result. Should I continue taking these tablets?

I usually advise *Thuja* tincture (ten drops twice daily) and I would be most surprised if that were to cause diarrhoea.

What would you recommend for rectal itching?
Dab the area twice daily with *Spilanthes* tincture and make sure that there is no *Candida* problem.

Could I have your views and advice on Alzheimer's disease?
It seems that often there is a link with aluminium toxicity, or possibly an allergic reaction to dental amalgam fillings. Both theories are being researched at present, but no definite verdict has been agreed. In some cases Chelation Therapy has proved helpful.

How can one reduce water retention in the tissues when on constant lithium salts medication (for manic depression)?
The best results I have obtained over the years were when my patients took 15 drops of Convascillan (before meals) and 15 drops of Hypericum (after meals), both twice daily.

Is there any help for senile dementia sufferers?
Sometimes Chelation Therapy can be beneficial although I have also had cases where I could not bring about any improvement in the condition. It is, however, always worth trying and the easiest remedy to use is oral chelation. You can read about it in my book *Heart and Blood Circulatory Problems*.

What can be done for genital herpes?
The Viraplex remedy is often helpful for this condition.

What would you advise for a failing memory?
Twice daily take 15 drops of *Ginkgo biloba* together with two Ginsavita tablets.

What can be done for a feeling of dizziness and a sensation of falling away?
Mostly I would suggest the remedy *Ginkgo biloba*. As I have recommended this remedy a number of times in this book I would like to say a little more about it here. *Ginkgo biloba* extract is currently attracting an enormous rise in popularity following extensive worldwide research, particularly in the area of its role in maintaining the circulation of blood to the brain. However, age researchers interested in mental performance are just one group of researchers working with the product, and many people believe

that in the next few years sales of *Ginkgo biloba* worldwide could outstrip those of most other plant extracts.

The *Ginkgo biloba* tree itself is a fascinating tree, being in effect a 'broad-leaved conifer'. It has remained largely unchanged for many centuries and its survival is being attributed to the fact that it has evolved an arsenal of potent chemicals with which it resists parasites, infections and pollution. These chemicals include flavonoid glycosides, flavonols, diterpenes and plant sterols. The leaves of the tree are the only part used and these are harvested when they are fully mature. It is at this time that the level of bioflavonoids is at its greatest. *Ginkgo* bioflavonoids have been shown to be up to ten times more effective at scavenging free radicals than other flavonoids. They are also thought to help maintain the circulation of blood to the brain and to the extremities of the body, such as the legs.

Why is complementary medicine not available on the NHS? Many people would like this who are at present unable to afford it.

It is indeed sad that people are expected to pay for remedies which are classified as alternative medicine. All I can say is keep applying pressure if you want to see this changed!

What can you advise for a person who always feels cold? Can this be a circulation problem? He is 65 years old.

If this person is always cold he should take 15 drops of Venosan together with five Urticalcin tablets twice daily.

What remedy would you suggest to make life bearable for people who live with an alcoholic?

Take two Neuroforce tablets twice daily.

What is the best source of natural energy for someone with sickle-cell anaemia?

Take four Alfalfa tablets each morning and night. Alfalfa, or lucerne, is a perennial herb that is found throughout continental Europe and is also cultivated in Britain. It contains small amounts of a wide variety of nutrients, especially trace elements, drawn from deep underground by exceptionally long tap roots, together with alkaloids and phytoestrogens.

I have had carpel tunnel syndrome for some time and a couple of months ago I had an operation. This has not been a

success and my fingers are still painful, as well as the wounds on my wrists. Because of the pain I cannot sleep. Any helpful advice would be appreciated.

I have seen great results with acupuncture treatment and usually I back this up with a zinc supplement.

Can you give me some advice for 'frozen shoulder'? I have suffered with this complaint for two years and despite having injections there has been no improvement.

A frozen shoulder can be very persistent and is usually caused by a minor injury or by bursitis or tendonitis. Even minimal movement can cause great pain. You should know that it ought to be treated as soon as possible or else this condition could become permanent. My suggestion would be acupuncture treatment and gentle manipulation. Using Imperthritica and Symphytum will also help.

I suffer badly from migraines and because of this I have started to grow feverfew, from which I make infusions. This helps and I would like your views on this.

This was an excellent decision. Feverfew has proved to be an effective remedy for migraines and headaches. This application is also mentioned in my book *Traditional Home and Herbal Remedies*.

What are the risks of contracting AIDS through acupuncture?

If the practitioner uses sterilised needles – as he or she should – there is no such risk. Personally, I find it easier to use disposable needles.

Could I please ask you about catarrh? Is it due to incorrect breathing, or environmental, dietary or a combination of factors?

Catarrh is often caused by a combination of influences. Enzymatic Therapy has developed a new remedy called AllerClear of which I have had good reports.

I have very dry skin, especially in winter, but I am allergic to many skin creams. Have you any recommendations?

The 7 Herb Cream from Dr Vogel is excellent and it is extremely unusual for users to experience any allergic reactions. *Symphytum* is also very good.

How would you treat nasal polyps?
Take 15 drops of *Marum verum* twice daily before meals.

How can we acquire the remedies you mention in your talks?
A list of useful addresses is given at the back of this book, as it is in all my books.

I have heard that you recommend *Marum verum* for snoring. How long will it take before it becomes effective?
Take 15 drops of *Marum verum* before meals and keep this up for 3–6 months.

How would you treat recurrent tonsillitis?
Take ten drops of Echinaforce twice daily.

What do you recommend to avoid hardening of the arteries?
You should adopt a healthy and balanced diet and take 15 drops of Arterioforce twice daily.

How would you treat a trapped nerve in the shoulder?
Usually by acupuncture and some osteopathic manipulation.

I am 69 years old and have suffered from mouth ulcers almost continually for the last twelve months. I have used the mouthwash recommended by my dentist and have also taken some New Era mineral tablets, but the ulcers still come back. They last for about one week and recur within days. I cannot think that they are diet-related because I take a very bland diet because of an oesophagal ulcer. I still have my own teeth and am puzzled as to the cause of this problem.
Your problem could be due to a sugar allergy and to find out if this is the case I suggest that you eliminate all sugar from your diet for a while. Take some supplementary vitamins, especially vitamin C, and twice a day use a mouthwash prepared with Molkosan (half a teaspoon mixed in half a cup of water).

Where can a test for mercury intolerance be done?
Any sympathetic dentist will be prepared to make the necessary arrangements for you.

I have alectasia, which means that I cannot digest milk sugars (lactose). Most antibiotics seem to contain lactose, which means that they make me very ill. I am due to have major dental surgery for which I will need antibiotics. My GP is wary of prescribing any antibiotics and I am asking you to advise me of what I could take.

A high dosage of Echinaforce will be of great help: take 30 drops before meals at least three times daily.

My husband has sudden sneezing bouts for no apparent reason. They can go on for some time and can be quite distressing. He can go for weeks without having an attack and they can happen at any time of the year. Have you any idea what could be the cause of these attacks?

Your description points towards an allergic reaction. My suggestion is that your husband takes 15 drops of Pollinosan before meals and 15 drops of *Harpagophytum* after meals, both twice daily.

What causes a coated tongue?

There can be various reasons for this, e.g. digestive causes or a liver indication. Try taking *Bryonia 6x*.

Seven years ago I had plastic surgery on my nose. The shape is not too bad, but the bone is permanently painful to the touch.

I am confident that acupuncture or laser therapy treatment would be of benefit.

If someone is allergic to shellfish, what would happen if they were to take the green-lipped mussel remedy?

You would be better advised not to use this remedy, because it is unlikely that it would agree with you.

I have a tic in my eyelid – what can I do?

Take two Neuroforce tablets twice daily.

Is there any remedy or treatment which would help confusion in the elderly?

Start immediately by taking 15 drops of *Ginkgo biloba* twice a day and you should soon notice an improvement.

Eight years ago I had a traumatic experience resulting in a burning tongue and gums. I have seen a consultant at the Dental Hospital and have had several new sets of dentures, but the problem is still with me. I would be so happy if you could help me in some way.

You would probably benefit from a *Propolis* supplement and could also try using a mouthwash made with half a teaspoon of Molkosan in half a glass of water. Use this mouthwash every day.

Can you possibly provide some advice for the spouse of an alcoholic who has become affected mentally, physically and spiritually by the disease?

You deserve all the understanding and sympathy you can get and you may find some useful information in my book *Stress and Nervous Disorders*.

How would you encourage a person to become well when his wife is constantly 'putting him down' with her negative remarks?

An open and honest talk between you and your partner with the help of a good marriage guidance counsellor would be the best course of action.

What have you to say about perfectionism?

There is nothing wrong with aiming for perfection so long as it is understood that other people's standards may not be as high as yours and so long as the striving for perfection does not become an obsession.

What can be done for 'mood swings'?

A positive outlook is required and for some extra help you could try taking 15 drops of *Zincum valerianicum* twice daily.

I sometimes fall asleep when driving in slow traffic, after meals or in a lecture. My memory and concentration also seems to be very poor. What can I do?

You should take great care and start immediately to take 15 drops of *Ginkgo biloba* together with two Ginsavita tablets.

My husband has been on painkillers since a motor accident some ten years ago. Our doctor says that he is addicted to them and we wondered if there is something else he could

take for the nerve pain and ulceration in the legs?
Natural painkillers are unlikely to become an addiction and I suggest that your husband tries taking two tablets of Petadolor twice daily. If this is not sufficiently effective I would further suggest that he consults an alternative practitioner, who will be able to offer more specific advice after he has examined your husband.

What is the cause of sebaceous cysts and what treatment would you recommend?
Sebaceous cysts are often caused by deficiencies, but can also be the result of infections. The treatment recommendation is to take ten drops of Petaforce twice daily.

What would be the best thing for phlegm?
Take 20 drops of Echinaforce twice daily.

My husband is 50 years old and over the last two years he has developed what he calls a 'cold nose'. Whenever the temperature changes his nose goes red and lately some red blood vessels are showing through. This is not alcohol-related.
You may rest assured that this is a fairly widespread problem. It is my experience that taking 15 drops of Venosan twice daily is very effective.

I am on an anti-cancer drug – Tamoxofam – and would like to know if it is possible to take natural remedies for another ailment alongside this?
There is no problem in taking natural remedies together with this drug.

Is there any cure for prickly heat? I have tried several homoeopathic remedies but they did not work and neither do anti-histamines. Can you think of anything that would ease the itch?
Twice a day take 15 drops of Nephrosolid in half a cup of Golden Grass Tea.

I have heard you speak about Nature's simple remedies. From some of my newspaper and magazine articles I have learned about people who follow the advice of some well-known

people, and who appear to be existing for weeks and even months on such restricted diets as lamb chops and pears, while taking doses of nystatin and large quantities of tablets containing all sorts of trace elements such as zinc, etc. What would you advise ME group members to do? Is it really as simple as you make out?

Of course, guidance is important and never more so than for what most people still consider the 'mysterious' illness ME. Coping with ME is not easy and therefore I greatly admire the work done by the numerous ME support groups.

Have you ever had any patients complain of the 'die-off phenomenon'? This is a very ill feeling while on an anti-fungal treatment. If you have heard of this before, please tell me how long I can expect this to last?

Fortunately, this symptom does not appear to be long-term. If you are experiencing this feeling you will benefit greatly if you take two Ginsavita tablets twice daily.

I have gout. What should I do?

People with gout are usually advised to avoid drinking alcohol. Also, ban from the diet red meat, fatty fish, chocolate and other rich foods. If you are a smoker you are strongly advised to stop. Take three 500 mg capsules of Oil of Evening Primrose last thing at night and 15 drops of Imperthritica twice daily.

What is thyroid eye disease?

Thyroid eye disease is an auto-immune condition. The term 'auto-immune' means that your own cells or antibodies are causing damage to certain of your body tissues. If you get a virus infection, your body produces a defence reaction which enables it to make antibodies to fight against the virus. In an auto-immune disease these same reactions are induced but instead of attacking a virus, they attack your own tissues. In the case of thyroid eye disease the attack is directed at the tissues at the back of the eye, including the muscles that control eye movements. This leads to inflammation and an increase of pressure behind the eye, so that the eye is sometimes pushed forward and may appear inflamed. The inflammation around the muscles at the back of the eye can sometimes result in double vision.

What is a hamstring?

Everyone has three hamstrings at the back of each leg. A hamstring is a tendon that is responsible for the bending of the knee or for the movement of the hip joint.

How many cranial nerves do we have?

There are 12 cranial nerves and most serve our sense organs, i.e. those responsible for sight, hearing, smell and taste. The longest cranial nerve is called the vagus nerve and this controls the parts of the body that move automatically, or involuntarily.

What is cranial osteopathy?

A cranial osteopath is specialised in working with the cranial nerves. Many ills can be rectified with the help of cranial osteopathy.

Is it normal for a woman to have lumps in her breast?

Whenever you detect any lump in your breast you should immediately have it checked by your doctor. There is no need to panic because most of the time there is no problem, but you would be wise to let your doctor decide. A woman's breast is made up of many glands that will produce milk during lactation. Like glands elsewhere in the body, these breast glands may swell occasionally. This often happens when breast-feeding, or during or prior to the monthly menstruation. A swelling may indicate a fibroid condition, also called fibroadenosis. It is, however, important to ask your doctor for an examination if and when you discover a change in your breasts.

I have stress incontinence and find this terribly embarrassing. Can you advise me?

Stress incontinence or leaking urine when coughing or laughing occurs when the muscles of the pelvic floor become weakened. These muscles control the bladder function. Exercises will help, as will 15 drops of Cystoforce taken twice daily.

What is Sjörgen's syndrome?

Sjörgen's syndrome is a disease in which the immune system attacks the salivary and tear (lachrymal) glands, leading to dryness of the eyes and mouth. It often causes fatigue and aching joints and muscles. An alternative practitioner will be able to prescribe specific remedies after examining the patient.

Glossary of remedies and suppliers

Acid phos.	Homoeopathic remedy
Acid picriam	Homoeopathic remedy
Acidophilus Plus	Nature's Best
Aconite	Homoeopathic remedy
Aesculaforce	Bioforce
Aesculus hipp.	Homoeopathic remedy
AkneZyme	Enzymatic Therapy
Alchemilla Complex	Bioforce
Alfavena	Bioforce
AllerClear	Enzymatic Therapy
Aloe Vera Cream	Nature's Best
Aluminia	Homoeopathic remedy
Amino Acid Chelate	Nature's Best
Apis mellificia	Homoeopathic remedy
Argentum nitricum	Homoeopathic remedy
ArMax	Enzymatic Therapy
Arnica	Bioforce
Arnica Ointment	A. Nelson
Arsenicum album	Bioforce
Arterioforce	Bioforce
ASM Drops	Bioforce
Avena sativa	Bioforce
Bambu	Bioforce
Belladonna	Bioforce
Berberis	Bioforce
Biodophilus	Nature's Best
Bioforce 7 Herb Cream	Bioforce
Boldocynara	Bioforce
Bronchosan	Bioforce

Byronia alba	Homoeopathic remedy
Calcara phos.	Homoeopathic remedy
Cantharis	Homoeopathic remedy
Carb. sulph.	Homoeopathic remedy
Cardiaforce	Bioforce
Centaurium	Bioforce
Cerebrum	Auchenkyle
Chelation Therapy	Auchenkyle
Chelidonium	Bioforce
China sulph.	Homoeopathic remedy
Cinnabaris	Bioforce
Coliacron	Auchenkyle
Coneflower Extract Capsules	Enzymatic Therapy
Conium mac.	Homoeopathic remedy
Convascillan	Auchenkyle
CoQ10	Nature's Best
CPS Formula	Enzymatic Therapy
Crataegus	Bioforce
Cystoforce	Bioforce
Detox Box Programme	Bioforce
Devil's Claw	Bioforce
DGL	Enzymatic Therapy
Diabetisan	Bioforce
Dioscorea	Homoeopathic remedy
Dormeasan	Bioforce
Drosinula Syrup	Bioforce
Echinacea Cream	Bioforce
Echinaforce	Bioforce
Euphrasia officinalis	Bioforce
Escalation Formula	Enzymatic Therapy
Femtrol	Enzymatic Therapy
Ferrum phos.	Homoeopathic remedy
Feverfew	Gerard House
FLW	Auchenkyle
Folic Acid	Nature's Best
Formula MGR417	Bioforce
Formula CPS	Enzymatic Therapy
Formula SNS	Bioforce

Fucus ves.	Homoeopathic remedy
Galeopsis	Bioforce
Gastronol	Bioforce
Gastrosan	Bioforce
GastroSoothe	Enzymatic Therapy
Gelsemium	Bioforce
Ginkgo biloba	Bioforce
Ginsavena	Bioforce
Ginsavita	Bioforce
Ginseng Capsules	Enzymatic Therapy
Golden Grass Tea	Bioforce
Graphites	Auchenkyle
GS500	Enzymatic Therapy
Gynovite Plus	Nature's Best
Hair and Skin Nutrition	Enzymatic Therapy
Hair Factor	Nature's Best
Hair Formula	Nature's Best
Hamamelis virg.	Bioforce
Harpagophytum	Bioforce
Health Insurance Plus	Nature's Best
Helianthus tuberosus	Bioforce
Hepar sulph.	Homoeopathic remedy
Herbamare	Bioforce
HiVitamin	Nature's Best
Hypericum	Bioforce
HypoAde	Enzymatic Therapy
Hyssop Tablets	Bioforce
Ignatia	Homoeopathic remedy
Imperthritica	Bioforce
Imuno-Strength	Nature's Best
Irish Moss	Healthfood Shop
Iron Plus	Nature's Best
Jan de Vries Health Tea	Auchenkyle
Jayvee Tablets	Nature's Best
Kalium iod.	Homoeopathic remedy
Kalium phos.	Homoeopathic remedy
Kava-Cara	Healthfood shops
Kelpasan	Bioforce

Lachesis	Bioforce
LGB Formula	Bioforce
Linoforce	Bioforce
Loranthus	Auchenkyle
Lycopodium virg.	Homoeopathic remedy
Lycopodus clav.	Homoeopathic remedy
Magnesium orotate	Gerard House
Marum verum	Bioforce
Masculex	Enzymatic Therapy
MegaZyme	Enzymatic Therapy
Melissa off.	Bioforce
Menopause Formula	Bioforce
Menosan	Bioforce
Merc. solub.	Homoeopathic remedy
Merzerium	Bioforce
MNP Formula	Bioforce
Molkosan	Bioforce
Migraine Formula	Bioforce
Myrtillis Complex	Healthfood shops
NaPCA Moisturiser	Nature's Best
Nat. mur.	Homoeopathic remedy
Nat. sulph.	Homoeopathic remedy
Nasturtium	Bioforce
Nephrosolid	Bioforce
Neuroforce	Bioforce
Nux vomica	Homoeopathic remedy
Oculosan	Bioforce
Onion Hair Lotion	Auchenkyle
Optivite	Nature's Best
Osteo-Balance	Nature's Best
Osteo-Care	Vitabiotics
OsteoPrime	Enzymatic Therapy
Ovarium	Bioforce
Ovasan	Bioforce
Pancreatin	Nature's Best
Papayasan	Bioforce
Passiflora	Bioforce
Peppermint Oil Capsules	Nature's Best

Peppermint Plus	Enzymatic Therapy
Perilla	Auchenkyle
Petaforce	Bioforce
Petasan	Bioforce
Pineapple Chews	Nature's Best
Plantaforce	Bioforce
Plantago majalis	Bioforce
PMS Formula	Bioforce
PoHo Oil	Bioforce
PoHo Ointment	Bioforce
Pollinosan	Bioforce
Priorin	Auchenkyle
Propolis	Healthfood shops
Propolis Gel	Auchenkyle
Prostabrit	Britannia Health Products
Prostasan	Bioforce
Psorinum	Homoeopathic remedy
Psoriasis Formula	Bioforce
Pulsatilla	Bioforce
Rasayana	Bioforce
Red Clover	Healthfood shops
RelaxoZyme	Enzymatic Therapy
Rescue Remedy	Bach Flower Remedies
Rheumarthaid Herb Box	Bioforce
Royal Gelee	Nature's Best
Rhumus	Homoeopathic remedy
Rhus tox.	Homoeopathic remedy
Sabal serr.	Homoeopathic remedy
Salvia	Bioforce
Salicylic Acid	Homoeopathic remedy
Santasapina	Bioforce
Seatone	Nature's Best
Selenium ACE	Healthfood shops
Sepia	Bioforce
Silicia	Homoeopathic remedy
Silymarin	Nature's Best
Solidago	Bioforce
Sinus Formula	Bioforce

SinuCheck	Enzymatic Therapy
Skin Formula	Vitabiotics
Skin Nutrition Capsules	Bioforce
Spigelia	Homoeopathic remedy
Spilanthes	Bioforce
St John's Wort Oil	Bioforce
Stinging Nettle Hair Lotion	Auchenkyle
Strophantus hisp.	Homoeopathic remedy
Sulphur	Homoeopathic remedy
Sulph. tid.	Homoeopathic remedy
Super Milk Thistle	Enzymatic Therapy
Symphytum officinalis	Bioforce
Symphytum Cream	Bioforce
Tabacum	Bioforce
Tanatia	Homoeopathic remedy
Taraxacum off.	Homoeopathic remedy
Temoe Lawak Tablets	Auchenkyle
Thuja	Homoeopathic remedy
Thymuplex	Enzymatic Therapy
Tormentavena	Bioforce
Toxeucal Oil	Bioforce
Tuberculinum	Homoeopathic remedy
Urticalcin	Bioforce
Usneasan	Bioforce
Valerian	Bioforce
Vasolastine	Auchenkyle
Venosan	Bioforce
Vinca Minor	Bioforce
Viola tricolor	Bioforce
Violaforce Cream	Bioforce
ViraPlex	Enzymatic Therapy
Vitalforce	Bioforce
Vogel's Slimming Formula	Bioforce
Zinc Citrate	Nature's Best
Zincum valerianicum	Homoeopathic remedy

USEFUL ADDRESSES

Auchenkyle
Southwoods Road
Troon
Ayrshire KA10 7EL

Bach Flower Remedies
Unit 6
Suffolk Way
Abingdon
Oxon OX14 5JX

Bioforce UK Ltd
Olympic Business Park
Dundonald
Ayrshire KA2 9BE

Bioforce USA Ltd
Kinderhook
New York
N.Y. USA

Britannia Health Products Ltd
Forum House
Brighton Road
Redhill
Surrey RH1 6YS

British Acupuncture Association
34 Alderney Street
London SW1V 4EU

Enzymatic Therapy
Hadley Wood Healthcare
67a Beech Hill
Hadley Wood
Barnet
Herts EN4 0JW

Enzymatic Therapy
P.O. Box 22310
Green Bay WI 54305
USA

General Council and Register of Naturopaths
Frazer House
6 Netherhall Gardens
London NW3 5RR

General Council and Register of Osteopaths
56 London Street
Reading
Berks RG1 4SQ

Gerard House
3 Wickham Road
Bournemouth
Dorset BH7 6JX

Nature's Best
1 Lamberts Road
Tunbridge Wells
Kent TN2 3EQ

A. Nelson & Co. Ltd
5 Endeavour Way
Wimbledon
London SW19 9UH

Vitabiotics Limited
Vitabiotics House
3 Bashley Road
London NW10 6SU